Saunders' Pocket Essentials of

General
Practice

Series Editors

Parveen Kumar and Michael Clark

Barts and the London, Queen Mary's School of
Medicine and Dentistry, University of London, UK

Commissioning Editor: Ellen Green
Development Editor: Ailsa Laing
Project Manager: Frances Affleck
Designer: Sarah Russell

Saunders' Pocket Essentials of

General Practice

Colin Bradley MD MICGP
Professor of General Practice, University College Cork,
Ireland

Series Editors
Parveen Kumar and **Michael Clark**

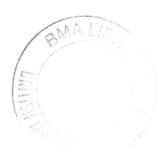

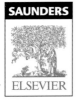

SAUNDERS

ELSEVIER

Edinburgh • London • New York • Oxford • Philadelphia •
St Louis • Sydney • Toronto 2006

SAUNDERS
ELSEVIER

An imprint of Elsevier Limited

ISBN 10: 0-7020-2648-4
ISBN 13: 978-0-7020-2648-5

British Library Cataloguing in Publication Data
A catalogue record for this book is available from the British Library

Library of Congress Cataloging in Publication Data
A catalog record for this book is available from the Library of Congress

Note
Neither the Publisher nor the Author assume any responsibility for any loss or injury and/or damage to persons or property arising out of or related to any use of the material contained in this book. It is the responsibility of the treating practitioner, relying on independent expertise and knowledge of the patient, to determine the best treatment and method of application for the patient.

The Publisher

Series Preface

Medical students and doctors in training are expected to travel to different hospitals and community health centres as part of their education. Many books are too large to carry on a regular basis, but are still necessary for the basic understanding of disease processes. This series of books is designed to provide portable, pocket-sized companions to larger texts such as *Clinical Medicine*. They all contain core material for quick revision, easy reference and practical management. The modern format makes them easy to read, providing an indispensable 'pocket essential'.

PJK
MLC

Preface

General practice has become a significant part of the curriculum of most medical schools. Yet there are still relatively few textbooks of general practice. This book aims to give a concise but broad overview of the discipline of general practice in a format that can fit in the pocket and, hence, be to hand when on attachment in general practice.

The first two chapters stress how general practice differs from hospital medicine with which most students are familiar. General practice is not just a cut down version of hospital medicine where there are fewer facilities for investigation and treatment of patients. The range of patients seen, the complaints with which they present, and the earlier stage of presentation mean that GPs have to approach the task of patient assessment quite differently. GPs must also try to manage all aspects of patient's diverse problems mostly within the constraints imposed by the community setting. The grouping of the detailed information on specific diseases and their management into chapters on emergencies, acute diseases and chronic diseases also reflects a somewhat different view of the clinical task when seen from the GP perspective. Remaining chapters pick up on other important aspects of general practice which have a particular or peculiar pertinence to general practitioners. Thus there are chapters on health promotion and prevention, on prescribing, on referral, and on the doctor–patient relationship. Like hospital doctors, GPs increasingly work in teams but our teams are quite different from those to be seen in hospital and these differences are covered on the chapter on the primary healthcare team. GPs occupy a unique position in the healthcare system and the features of different healthcare systems impinge on GPs more so than they do on many other doctors. The current positions of British and Irish GPs in their distinct health systems are outlined to help students understand the importance of the health system to GPs and vice versa. Finally, ethical issues challenge all doctors but some of the ethical issues challenging GPs are quite distinctive and subtle as is explained in the final chapter.

While many purely clinical questions arising in general practice can be addressed by knowledge arising from other disciplines such as medicine, surgery, paediatrics, psychiatry, and so forth the application of this knowledge in a general practice setting is distinctive. Other issues are particular to general practice – such as questions of whom to refer and when. General practitioners are also focused more on the people who present to them with diseases (or perceived diseases) than on the diseases these people have. 'Person centred' medicine is particularly evident in general practice. GPs meet the challenges involved in trying to help their patients with different resources available in the community. Attachments in general practice are aimed at helping students appreciate all these specific features of general practice while also capitalising on the rich environment general practice presents for acquiring knowledge and understanding of all branches of medicine. It is hoped this book can be an informative and practical guide for students encountering the rich clinical learning environment that is general practice.

Contents

1

The nature and scope of general practice

General practice

Specialist medical disciplines tend to be described in terms of either the body system to which they relate (e.g. cardiology) or the age group of patients to whom they relate (e.g. paediatrics). General practice is a generalist discipline not confined to any one body system or group of patients, although in some countries specific groups of patients, such as children, may be looked after by community-based specialists such as paediatricians. To clarify the boundaries of the discipline of general practice WONCA Europe (Box 1.1) has provided:

- a definition of the discipline of general practice/family medicine
- a description of the specialty of general practice/family medicine

Box 1.1   WONCA

WONCA is an acronym for the World Organization of National Colleges, Academies and Academic Associations of General Practitioners/Family Physicians, or World Organization of Family Doctors for short.
www.globalfamilydoctor.com

- a statement of the core competencies required of family doctors.

According to WONCA general practice/family medicine is an academic and scientific discipline, with its own educational content, research, evidence base and clinical activity, and a clinical specialty orientated to primary care.

Definition of the discipline

The 11 central characteristics of the discipline of general practice/family medicine are that it:

1. is normally the point of first medical contact within the healthcare system, providing open and unlimited access to its users, dealing with all health problems regardless of the age, sex, or any other characteristic of the person concerned.
2. makes efficient use of healthcare resources through co-ordinating care, working with other professionals in the primary care setting, and managing the interface with other specialties, taking an advocacy role for the patient when needed.
3. develops a person-centred approach, orientated to the individual, his/her family, and their community.
4. has a unique consultation process, which establishes a relationship over time, through effective communication between doctor and patient.
5. is responsible for the provision of longitudinal continuity of care, as determined by the needs of the patient.
6. has a specific decision-making process determined by the prevalence and incidence of illness in the community.

7. manages simultaneously both acute and chronic health problems of individual patients.
8. manages illness that presents in an undifferentiated way at an early stage in its development, which may require urgent intervention.
9. promotes health and wellbeing by appropriate and effective intervention.
10. has a specific responsibility for the health of the community.
11. deals with health problems in their physical, psychological, social, cultural and existential dimensions.

Description of the specialty

General practitioners/family doctors are specialist physicians trained in the principles of the discipline. They are personal doctors, primarily responsible for the provision of comprehensive and continuing care to every individual seeking medical care, irrespective of age, sex and illness. They care for individuals in the context of their family, their community and their culture, always respecting the autonomy of their patients. They also have a professional responsibility to their community. In negotiating management plans with their patients they integrate physical, psychological, social, cultural and existential factors, utilising the knowledge and trust engendered by repeated contacts.

General practitioners/family physicians exercise their professional role by promoting health, preventing disease and providing cure, care, or palliation. This is done either directly or through the services of others, according to health needs and the resources available within the community they serve, assisting patients where necessary in accessing these services. They must take responsibility for developing and maintaining their skills, personal balance and values as a basis for effective and safe patient care.

The core competencies

A definition of the discipline, and of the specialist family doctor, must lead directly to the core competencies. Core means essential to the discipline, irrespective of the healthcare system in which they are applied. The 11 central characteristics that define the discipline (relating to the 11 abilities that every specialist family doctor should master, listed above) can be clustered into six core competencies:

- primary care management (1, 2)
- person-centred care (3, 4, 5)
- specific problem-solving skills (6, 7)
- comprehensive approach (8, 9)
- community orientation (10)
- holistic modelling (11).

To practise the specialty the competent practitioner implements these competencies in three areas:

- clinical tasks
- communication with patients
- management of the practice.

As a person-centred scientific discipline, three background features should be considered as fundamental:

- contextual: using the context of the person, the family, the community and their culture
- attitudinal: based on the doctor's professional capabilities, values and ethics
- scientific: adopting a critical and research-based approach to practice and maintaining this through continuing learning and quality improvement.

The interrelation of core competencies, implementation areas and fundamental features characterises the discipline and underlines the complexity of the specialty. It is this complex interrelationship of core competencies that should guide and be reflected in the development of related agendas for teaching, research and quality improvement.

The full definition and the accompanying commentary are available at the WONCA Europe website (see Further Reading).

Definition of general practice

In common with most, the WONCA definition emphasises the six core competencies outlined above.

Primary care

Primary care is the first point of contact between a patient and the health service. First-contact care occurs elsewhere in the health services (e.g. in Accident and Emergency departments), but is a much more significant part of the GP's work. This does not mean that the GP has to deal with all problems presented, indeed, it is an essential requirement of good GPs to know the limitations of their skills and remit, and how and when to refer or delegate (see Chapter 8).

Primary care also involves working with others in a non-hierarchical fashion (see Chapter 10). Holistic care (see below) works best when the team is non-hierarchical. Hierarchical teams, such as operate in the hospital setting, are not necessary in the community setting and are inappropriately dehumanising.

Finally, primary care physicians are required to mediate between patients and other levels of the health and social care systems, which requires doctors to act as advocates for their patients upon occasion.

Personal and continuing care

A GP is ideally seen as someone the patient can identify as 'my doctor'. The relationship between patient and GP is usually a long-term one built on mutual respect and trust (see Chapter 9). The relationship may span large parts of the patient's lifetime, including episodes of illness where care is shared with specialists. While specialists also provide on-going care, this usually relates only to that part of the care of the patient that falls within their specialist domain. GPs provide ongoing care to all types of patient, including psychological and social care (see Chapter 5).

Specific problem-solving skills

All problems presented by patients require a response on the part of the doctor. While the GP may not be able to resolve all problems, each will require some form of decision. This may be a decision that no further action is required, a decision to instigate a treatment in general practice or a decision to refer to other source(s) of help – or any combination of these. GPs also deploy specific diagnostic and management styles that differ from those in specialist practice (see Chapter 2).

Comprehensive approach

GPs have obligations to patients, particularly those who adopt them as their personal or family physician, that go beyond providing a response to symptoms or problems presented. They also have obligations to provide preventive healthcare measures and to promote patients' health more generally (see Chapter 6). The range of interventions available to the GP need not, and ought not to, be confined to the purely therapeutic (i.e. drugs, surgery, etc.).

Family and community orientation

A GP will very often be physician to several, or sometimes all, members of a family. In many parts of the world the term 'family doctor' is used to refer to what we call a GP. General practice is sometimes called 'family medicine' or 'family practice'. The concept of a family doctor has been eroded, to an extent, by changes in society – particularly the move away from large extended families living in close proximity toward nuclear families and persons living alone. However, there are still many opportunities to gain valuable insights into people and their problems from knowledge of the family background.

On a biological level the diagnosis of genetically determined health problems may be facilitated by knowing the hereditary diseases that have afflicted other members of the family. On a sociological level the knowledge of one family member's social situation or illness behaviour may help understand how, when or why another family member chooses to attend the GP.

Holistic modelling

It is recognised that patients, particularly where they have unrestricted access to a doctor for any problem, will bring in all sorts of problems – including many which are not strictly medical. To deal with these effectively the GP needs to be alert to the psychological and social genesis of symptoms. More importantly, though, patients' problems are usually multifaceted with physical, psychological and social components, all of which should be acknowledged – even when a judgement will be required as to which one predominates and requires active management. This is the holistic nature of care that GPs aim to provide.

Not all aspects of this definition are accepted by all commentators on general practice as necessary in order to allow use of the term 'GP' or 'family doctor'. Other terms, such as primary care physician, office-based physician/internist and community doctor, may be used to describe doctors who accept many but not all aspects of this definition. There are also disagreements regarding the relative importance of these features in determining whether or not a doctor is really a GP or some other form of primary care/community based physician.

Some features of the definition vary in their manifestation from healthcare system to healthcare system and some aspects of the definition are quite aspirational.

Differences from hospital medicine

For medical students who are already familiar with hospital medicine, a consideration of how general practice medicine differs from this is a useful way of coming to an understanding of general practice. There are four main differences:

- the variety and nature of health problems seen
- how these are dealt with or managed
- the nature of the relationships (both doctor–patient relationships and relationships between healthcare professionals)

- how it is organised – both administratively and in terms of physical infrastructure.

The nature of illnesses seen

Table 1.1 illustrates the contrasts between general practice medicine and hospital medicine in terms of the illnesses seen.

Unorganised illness and non-disease

By the time patients arrive at hospital they will often have some inkling as to the nature of the condition. Patients on cardiology wards usually have cardiac problems and patients in mental health centres usually have psychiatric problems. On arrival to the GP the patient may have a constellation of symptoms, which may or may not fit into

Table 1.1
Contrast between general practice and hospital medicine in terms of the illnesses seen

General practice	Hospital
Unorganised illness and non-disease (i.e. symptoms without underlying disease)	Mostly clear-cut diseases
Acute presentations usually benign and self-limiting	Acute presentations often life-threatening
Chronic illnesses mostly in a stable phase	Chronic illnesses usually in unstable phase (acute-on-chronic)
Patients of all ages	Patients may be categorised by age particularly young (paediatrics) and old (geriatrics)
Patients not usually categorised by illness type	Patients usually categorised by illness type
Mixed physical, psychological and social problems, often co-existing in same patient; all elements of problem explicitly acknowledged	Problems and patients categorised as either physical or psychological – social problems only rarely acknowledged as the principal reason for attendance/admission

8

patterns associated with one or other body system or one or other particular disease.

All symptoms are given equal weight by the patient in what is called 'unorganised illness'. The GP interprets the patient's story, placing emphasis on those features that might be associated with identifiable diseases while paying less attention to those that do not fit a typical clinical syndrome. Thus, the next time the patient explains the symptoms, the story may become more 'organised' with some initial symptoms played down or omitted. 'Non-disease' is a name given to symptoms that turn out, in the end, to have no particular disease associated with them.

Acute presentations of benign self-limiting disease

Partly as a consequence of being a point of first contact with the healthcare system, GPs will see a much greater proportion of symptoms that signify only minor self-limiting health problems (see Chapter 4). This high proportion of patients with benign self-limiting diseases accounting for their symptoms presents the GP with several challenges:

- to rule out possible serious causes for the patient's symptoms
- to discover what underlies the patient's decision to consult (usually an anxiety about a possible serious illness or for some specific treatment or help)
- to explain the benign nature of the patient's condition and yet avoid 'medicalising' the problem
- to manage time so as to give enough attention to all patients and yet not spend too much time dealing with minor problems that do not particularly require a GP's effort or skills
- to encourage self-management.

Chronic illness

As the population ages and more people survive to old age as the result of earlier medical interventions, the number of people living with long-term health problems will increase. Furthermore, as acute life-threatening illnesses become increasingly rare, the proportion of doctors' work taken up with looking after the chronically ill increases. The GPs role in the management of people with chronic disease tends to involve monitoring the patient during periods of relative stability rather than necessarily dealing with acute phases of the chronic illness, although this will vary from disease to disease (see Chapter 5). The GP will also often have to deal with the psychological and social effects of a patient's long-term illness on both the patient and the family.

Patients of all ages, genders and illness type

In hospital patients are often segregated according to their age – children will be looked after by paediatricians, the very old by specialists in healthcare of the elderly. Adults will usually be segregated according to the presumed nature of their complaint and sometimes by gender. In general practice there are no such barriers. In some countries, though, children will be seen by office-based paediatricians, adults by a variety of office-based specialists in lieu of general practitioners.

Physical, psychological and social problems

A very important concept that has greatly influenced the development of general practice as an academic discipline is that of the multidimensional nature of patients' problems. Sometimes referred to as the bio-psycho-social model or as the tri-axial concept, this recognises that patients' problems all have a physical, a psychological and a social dimension. One of the requirements of a GP is to judge which of these dimensions is the most important and the one where interventions might help resolve the problem. In hospital patients will be categorised into those whose problem is judged to be mainly physical or mainly psychological. Social problems in hospital patients are not usually acknowledged as the reason for hospitalisation and are not the focus of doctors' attention.

Recognising the multidimensional nature of patients' problems also impinges on management. Ideally, all aspects of the problem should be addressed in the management of the patient. Thus, as well as treating the physical symptoms of a respiratory tract infection (physical dimension) a GP may be expected to allay fears about other causes (psychological dimension) and provide a sickness certificate to excuse the patient from work (social dimension).

Organisation

Table 1.2 illustrates the contrasts between general practice medicine and hospital medicine in terms of their organisation.

Size of unit

General practices are small units with staff numbers not usually exceeding 50 in total (and often very much fewer), including medical and non-medical staff. They are housed in premises usually of a few thousand square feet. They are non-institutionalised, with patients and staff often knowing each other quite well. While there will be rhythm and routine, the pattern of work is generally fairly flexible, with staff often working and taking breaks as demands allow rather than to a strict timetable and everyone helping out, perhaps regardless of strict role definition.

Hospitals are, by contrast, large capital-intensive units with staff numbers in the hundreds or even thousands and in large buildings of tens of thousands of square feet. People

Table 1.2
Contrast between general practice and hospital medicine in terms of their organisation

General practice	Hospital
Small units, non-institutionalised	Large institutional units
Non-hierarchical teams	Highly hierarchical teams
Low tech	High tech
Easily accessible	Filtered access

will tend to work in sub-units where they may know each other but it will not always be possible for staff to know all the other people working in the institution. Roles tend to be strictly defined and strictly adhered to. Work for many in a hospital setting is scheduled according to quite rigid timetables.

Hierarchical and non-hierarchical teams

Teamwork plays an important part in both hospital and general practice but the nature of the teams differs. In hospitals there are several teams – a medical team, a nursing team and so on – each with their own hierarchy. These teams co-operate in well worked out routines, which allow each team to make its distinct contribution to patient care. Within each team there is a hierarchy that makes it clear who has the power to make what decisions. This is all necessary in the intensive working situation that characterises hospitals, where the room for error is potentially quite large and the consequences of error quite great. Strict hierarchies and role definitions reduce the risk of error.

In general practice there is less need for hierarchies and a greater need for staff to be flexible. A more egalitarian structure makes for easier communication as situations evolve and for wider ranges of solutions to be considered. This is necessary because of the nature of general practice problems (see above). They are often complex, multifaceted problems with no one optimal solution. Thus, for example, if you have acute appendicitis there is only one correct way to proceed and that is to have your appendix removed, ideally by a competent team of surgeons assisted in a prescribed manner by equally competent nurses all following a well worked out routine.

If you have multiple respiratory tract infections and low mood as a consequence of working in a dirty environment and living in poor housing in a rundown area, no one member of the team will have all the answers to your problems. Each team member needs to be capable of thinking laterally and the team must be able to brainstorm to come up with possible solutions to improve your lot.

Low tech versus high tech

Part of the rationale for concentrating healthcare in large institutions like hospitals is to gain the economies of scale that can justify the investment of relatively large sums of money required for the high tech equipment now used in hospitals. General practice, by contrast, has less need for high tech equipment and relies on lower tech equipment for making diagnoses and managing patients. This is changing as technology of an appropriate size and cost become available which allows the GP to do more diagnosis and management 'in house'. There was a time when a GP's diagnostic equipment would consist of a thermometer, a stethoscope, a sphygmomanometer, an otoscope and an ophthalmoscope. Now most GPs will use peak flow meters, ECG machines, autoclaves and an ever-increasing array of new patient tests in their practices.

Ease of access

As has been stressed above, one of the defining characteristics of general practice is the ease of access for patients – it acts as the most frequently accessed point of first contact with the health service. Access to hospitals, with the exceptions of Accident and Emergency departments and Genitourinary Medicine (formerly STD) clinics, is generally limited by the requirement for patients to be referred by their general practitioner. This filtering of access to hospital by GPs is referred to as the 'gate-keeper' function (see Chapter 8).

Common conditions seen

In terms of the physical illnesses seen in general practice, the categories of illness are broadly similar to those seen in hospital. Thus GPs will see illnesses from all the major systems – cardiovascular, respiratory, digestive system etc. However, the proportions of patient contacts involving these types of condition will differ slightly (Table 1.3). What

Table 1.3
Proportions of patients seen in general practice and hospital, by selected ICD (International Classification of Disease) categories

ICD heading	General practice	Hospital
Infection	4%	2%
Neoplasms	1%	8%
Mental disorders	10%	4%
Cardiovascular	8%	9%
Respiratory	19%	8%
Digestive	4%	10%
Genitourinary	5%	8%
Childbirth & pregnancy	10%	19%
Skin conditions	6%	2%
Musculoskeletal	7%	3%
Symptoms and ill-defined conditions	8%	6%
Accidents	5%	10%

From National Morbidity survey and Hospital Episode statistics compiled by the NHS Health and Social Care Information Centre.

is more significant, though, is the nature of the illnesses seen within these categories. Thus, for example, COPD and asthma are common in both settings but diseases that are rare in hospital (e.g. sarcoidosis) will be very rare in general practice and there will be a range of common diseases, such as cold and 'flu, which will be seen a lot in general practice and rarely, if at all, in hospital. Table 1.4 lists the common physical illnesses seen in general practice by system and Table 1.5 lists some common psychological and social problems seen.

As well as physical illnesses, general practitioners will see many psychological problems (some co-existing with physical illnesses) and a number of social problems. In contrast to physical problems, these psychological and social problems can be quite serious but managing them may be more challenging as there are fewer clear-cut solutions for many of them, particularly social problems. Even where there are potential solutions the resources required to provide these are often less readily available.

Table 1.4
Some common illnesses in general practice by system

System	Common illnesses
Respiratory	Colds, influenza, asthma, bronchitis
Gastrointestinal	Gastroenteritis, peptic ulcer disease, irritable bowel syndrome
Cardiovascular	Hypertension, ischaemic heart disease
Musculoskeletal	Back pain, osteoarthritis, soft tissue injury
Endocrine	Diabetes, thyroid disease
Genitourinary	Urinary tract infection, sexually transmitted infections, dysfunctional uterine bleeding
Skin conditions	Eczema, psoriasis, skin infections

Table1.5
Common psychological and social problems in general practice

Type of problem	Common examples
Psychological	Adjustment reactions e.g. grief
	Anxiety
	Depression
	Mixed anxiety and depression
	Drug and alcohol problems
	Chronic stable schizophrenia
	Post-traumatic stress disorder
Social problems	Relationship difficulties
	Job dissatisfaction
	Effects of poor housing
	Effects of unemployment
	Effects of social deprivation
	Lack of education

Specialism versus generalism

One of the most important differences to appreciate between general practice and other medical disciplines is that general practice is not another specialism – it is unique in being a generalist discipline. In other branches of medicine progress is usually associated with an ever more refined and detailed knowledge and understanding of disease processes and the techniques used in their management. This vast burden of knowledge cannot be effectively retained by single individuals, so individuals confine themselves to smaller and smaller areas of expertise in order to be able to keep up effectively. This reductionist approach to knowledge leads to ever more sub-sub-specialism. This has many advantages, not least that the sub-sub-specialist will know virtually everything to be known in one area – but at the cost of knowing little of anything else.

While the ever-greater specialism of medicine has brought considerable benefits it is, paradoxically dependent on a cadre of generalists who know enough of all the different sub-specialties to ensure that people end up under the care of the appropriate specialist. Thus the growth of specialism makes the need for generalists greater rather than less (see also Chapter 8). The generalist's key skills are in knowing enough of everything to ensure:

- that those whose problem is not sufficiently difficult or severe as to need specialist intervention are not unnecessarily referred
- that those who do need specialist attention receive it.

Further reading

European Definition of General Practice/Family Medicine. WONCA Europe http://www.medisin.ntnu.no/wonca/
Fry J, Sandler G 1993 Common diseases: their nature, prevalence and care. Kluwers Academic, Dordrecht, The Netherlands
McWhinney I R 2004 A textbook of family medicine, 2nd edn. Oxford University Press, Oxford

Approach to diagnosis and treatment

General practice shares with other branches of medicine the tasks of diagnosing and managing the patient's health problems. However, being based in the community, the number of patients seen each day, the nature of the problems presented, the lack of high tech diagnostic tools and the lack of expertise in, and access to, certain forms of treatment mean that the GP has to adapt the approach to these tasks to take account of these constraints. That said, the adaptations, such as an efficient approach to diagnosis and a multi-faceted approach to management, are techniques that can be useful to any doctor regardless of the work setting.

Diagnosis

Three distinct approaches to the task of diagnosis or identifying the nature of the patient's problem are described:

- the inductive approach
- the hypothetico-deductive approach
- pattern recognition.

The inductive approach

This is the approach usually taught first to medical students. It has parallels with the inductive approach to acquiring knowledge in general. The procedure, amply described in textbooks of clinical method, is often referred to as 'doing a complete history and physical'. It comprises collection of data from the patient on:

- the presenting complaint
- the history of the presenting complaint
- past medical, surgical and psychiatric history
- drug history (including history of any allergies)
- systems inquiry comprising questions about all the common symptoms associated with each bodily system
- social history including tobacco and alcohol consumption.

This is followed by a complete physical examination of all systems of the body.

In the inductive approach all this data is gathered before generating a principal diagnosis or possibly a list of differential diagnoses, which are then tested by means of specific investigations.

The hypothetico-deductive approach

An alternative approach is one that parallels the hypothetico-deductive approach of modern scientific inquiry in which observations are made, hypotheses are generated and then tested in the light of new observations often derived from specific experiments set up to test the hypothesis.

In this clinical method the initial presentation of the patient (including age, gender etc.), presenting complaint and any other immediately obvious facts (such as showing signs of distress) or background information known to the physician (such as having had similar symptoms before) immediately give rise to some preliminary ideas or hypotheses regarding the diagnosis. By means of selective enquiries and examination of the patient the doctor seeks to test these diagnostic ideas, eventually coming up with the one that is most probable or with a strategy using further tests to narrow the range of possibilities to one that will be sufficiently probable to guide future management (Fig. 2.1). Studies of the diagnostic thinking of doctors in real life situations suggests that this is how most diagnoses are actually made.

Pattern recognition
A further route to diagnosis is 'pattern recognition'. In this approach the presenting features of the case are so strongly

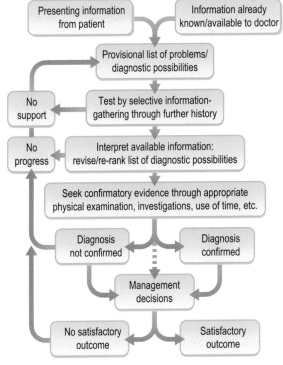

Fig. 2.1 **The hypothetico-deductive approach to diagnosis.**

suggestive of only one possible diagnosis that the doctor immediately recognises this. For example, one look at a miserable child with a cough, temperature, running eyes and nose and the characteristic rash can be enough to tell the experienced clinician that the child has measles. Further history taking and examination serve only to confirm what the doctor already 'knows'. Pattern recognition is, arguably, a variant of the hypothetico-deductive approach in which only one diagnosis is considered and all the evidence needed for testing this is immediately apparent.

Advantages and disadvantages of the different approaches

In clinical practice a mixture of three approaches to diagnosis is used (Table 2.1). Where there are features that fit an easily recognised condition in a very reliable and predictable way doctors may rely on pattern recognition – with the proviso to the patient to reconsult if things do not progress as expected (see 'safety netting' p. 27). More typically GPs will use hypothetico-deductive thinking when a few likely possibilities suggest themselves. Where no hypothesis suggests itself (an uncommon situation for the experienced practitioner but more common for the novice) a systematic inductive approach is used, maybe reverting to a hypothesis-testing mode if a possible diagnosis begins to emerge.

Factors that influence the possibilities

There are four main influences on the diagnoses generated in the hypothetico-deductive approach:

- probability
- seriousness
- treatability
- novelty.

Probable diagnoses are the most likely to account for the patient's symptoms. However, other possible diagnoses – which, while less probable, are very serious if true – must also be considered. Knowing which conditions are probable

Table 2.1
Advantages and disadvantages of different approaches to diagnosis

Approach	Advantages	Disadvantages
Inductive	Suitable for students (with limited knowledge of diseases) Allows data gathering without the need for prior hypothesis generation Enables skills of history taking and examination to be honed Useful for generation of hypotheses when hypothetico-deductive approach fails Done properly, all the relevant facts will be gathered in the end; reduces risk of overlooking important facts Minimises risk of overlooking diagnostic possibilities	Time consuming (30 mins minimum) The more complex the patient's problem the longer it takes Tedious for patient and doctor May generate too much data Information overload Too many possibilities to be explored Not very intuitive Cannot really stop people hypothesising before all the data is gathered
Hypothetico-deductive	Matches our intuitive problem-solving approach Often successful Avoids information overload Quick, efficient and usually effective (average 10 mins to reach a diagnosis)	Error prone, especially for inexperienced or those lacking knowledge of disease More likely to lead to missing a rare diagnosis or multiple diagnoses Requires doctor to generate reasonable diagnoses quickly Requires good knowledge and experience of likely possibilities and their presenting features Need to know most effective questions to ask to get quick responses
Pattern recognition	Quick and easy	Very error prone, especially if inexperienced Only suitable for a very limited range of diagnoses with very specific clinical features

requires knowledge of the epidemiology of different conditions in the context in which each case is seen and in the
different ages, genders, etc. of patients. This can be illustrated in the case of patients presenting with cough. Figure
2.2 shows the distribution of the likely causes of coughs
according to their duration. Figure 2.3 shows how the probability of different causes of cough varies with the age of the
patient.

Knowing which conditions are serious comes of having
knowledge of the markers of serious illness (e.g. abnormal
vital signs) and having seen the more serious end of the

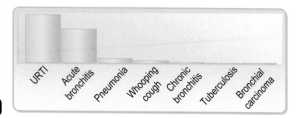

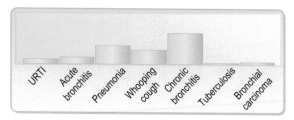

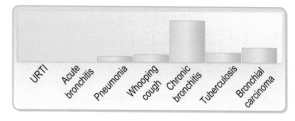

Fig. 2.2 **Likelihood of different causes of cough of (a) 3 days
duration, (b) 3 weeks duration, and (c) 3 months duration.**

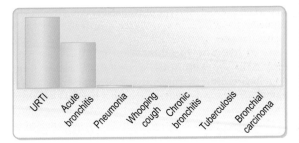

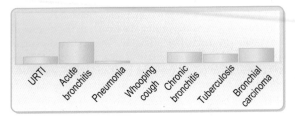

Fig. 2.3 **Likelihood of different causes of cough in (a) a 3-year-old child, and (b) a 70-year-old.**

disease spectrum in hospital. This combination of probable and serious diagnostic possibilities should be used to determine the list of diagnoses to be tested in the hypothetico-deductive process. However, there is a tendency for doctors to consider more actively diagnoses for which there is an effective treatment, overlooking conditions lacking such a treatment. This might seem to be of little consequence given that a diagnosis of an untreatable condition will be of little benefit to the patient. However, an untreatable diagnosis being overlooked may lead to a treatable condition being erroneously diagnosed instead and wrong or unhelpful treatment being instigated.

Finally, one other factor known to influence diagnostic thinking has been described as 'novelty'. This refers to a new or unfamiliar diagnosis being attributed to the patient's symptoms because the doctor has just heard of it or seen it turn up unexpectedly in another patient. While it is important to avoid this type of availability error, this can be difficult.

Aids to hypothesis generation

One of the key skills in the successful application of the hypothetico-deductive method is generating enough relevant diagnostic possibilities – the other being to test these properly. Diseases can be classified according to the nature of the disease process, according to the system affected or according to the predominant dimension of the problem. All of these can be used as schema to generate hypotheses about the likely cause of a patient's symptoms (Table 2.2).

The use of schema regarding the nature of the disease or the system affected is quite straightforward. The bio-psycho-social schema is more specific to general practice. All illness has physical/biological, psychological and sociological components. However, when it comes to managing the patient's problem GPs usually have to decide which component or components of the illness they are going to be able to help with. Categorising the problem as primarily physical, psychological or social can be used as an aid to hypothesis generation. For example, if a patient presents with feeling 'tired all the time' likely physical causes would include anaemia, thyroid disease, diabetes etc. Psychological causes could include anxiety or depression, while overwork, job

Table 2.2
Classification of diseases by differing criteria

Disease process	System	Bio-psycho-social
Congenital	Cardiovascular	Physical
Acquired	Respiratory	Psychological
– Traumatic	Gastrointestinal	Social
– Infective	Genitourinary	
– Inflammatory	Musculoskeletal	
– Metabolic	Neurological	
– Neoplastic	Dermatological	
– Haemopoietic	Haematological	
– Psychogenic	Psychiatric	
– Iatrogenic		

stress or irregular sleep habits could be possible social causes.

Types of hypotheses generated by GPs

The above discussion might suggest that the main diagnostic task of GPs is to ascribe the patient's problem to some sort of diagnostic category, such as would be recognised by any other doctor. While this is certainly part of what is required, it is only one factor. GPs need to be able to formulate ideas on a range of aspects of the patient's problem. Before even assigning it to a disease category or giving it a disease label, the GP may have to decide what sort of a problem the patient has. It may not be a medical problem, or at least not exclusively. A judgement needs to be made with regard to which aspects of the problem – physical, psychological, or social – merit the greatest attention.

The GP also needs to formulate ideas on how the patient is responding to the problem. What does the patient think is the matter? What about the problem concerns the patient? Are their specific or general fears about the condition and/or its possible consequences? What is it the patient hopes or expects the doctor to do about the problem? Thus GPs do not make singular diagnoses but rather come to a range of diagnostic hypotheses about the patient and the problem.

Testing diagnostic possibilities

Having generated a range of possible diagnoses to account for the patient's presenting complaints, these need to be tested by further history taking and examination. The patient's history is acquired in the course of a doctor–patient encounter or consultation (see Chapter 9). The aim of achieving a diagnosis is served by gathering information that helps to either 'rule out' (by revealing the absence of symptoms) or 'rule in' a possible diagnosis (by the presence of symptoms).

This concept of diagnosis involving either ruling in or ruling out disease is an application of Bayes' Theorem

(Box 2.1). Major implications following from this important concept are:

- In making diagnoses we are strongly influenced by our prior beliefs (which are really just probabilistic judgements) regarding what are likely causes for the patient's problems.
- All information we receive (through history taking, examination, or investigations) shifts the probabilities of different diagnoses towards making them more likely or less likely explanations of the patient's presentation.
- The effectiveness of any given test (which could include questions asked of a patient or a clinical finding on examination) depends critically on the difference between prior probabilities and posterior probabilities.
- These probabilities, in turn, are critically dependent on:
  - the characteristics of the test (i.e. sensitivity and specificity)
  - the prevalence of the condition of interest in the population.

Sensitive tests are generally good for ruling disease out and specific tests are good for ruling disease in. For a fuller discussion of the issues involved in making diagnoses based on how probabilities of diagnoses are affected by characteristics of the disease, the test and the population in which

---

Box 2.1 **Bayes' Theorem**

Bayes' Theorem is a mathematical principle that states that the probability of a hypothesis being true given that we have made some observations (called the 'posterior probability') is a function of the probability you would have assigned to the hypothesis prior to making the observations (the 'prior probability') and the probabilities of the observations occurring if the hypothesis were true and the probability of the observations occurring if the hypothesis were false.

the diagnosis is being attempted, readers should consult textbooks of clinical epidemiology or evidence-based medicine.

In general practice the position is more often of ruling out serious diagnoses, which is best achieved by demonstrating the absence of key expected features associated with serious diseases. Ruling in diagnoses requires more specific confirmatory tests, which are more often available in hospital than in general practice. Furthermore, ruling in benign diseases may be more difficult as they do not often produce specific clinical signs. Even if there are laboratory investigations that might establish a specific disease, where the disease is likely to be of limited clinical significance it will not be worth doing the test (see also Chapter 4).

Safety netting

'Safety netting' is the name given to the strategies used by GPs to try and ensure that, if their diagnosis is not correct, any potential harm to the patient will be minimised. Typically, this will be simple techniques such as routinely telling patients to come back or make further contact if they are not happy with the progress of their illness. Sometimes, more explicit or precise instructions may be given, e.g. asking the parent of an ill child to ring back after several hours and report on progress when the child appears to have a simple viral infection but a more serious condition, such as early stage meningitis, cannot be confidently excluded. Sometimes patients are given a prescription but asked only to fill it if the condition worsens. This practice is called 'deferred prescribing'.

When giving instructions to patients for the purposes of safety netting, they should be as clear as possible. Providing the patient with objective indicators, such as a certain rise in temperature, the appearance of any ominous symptoms or the persistence of symptoms beyond a certain time frame, is very helpful to patients and ensures effective safety netting.

Management options

While GPs might be seen as having a restricted range of treatment options available compared with hospital colleagues, this is not entirely true. Certainly, in hospital patients can be treated with a wider variety of drugs and there is a range of surgical and quasi-surgical therapeutic procedures (such as angioplasty). However, these are not necessarily the kinds of interventions required by patients presenting to GPs – the problem may be very minor or may be one that is not strictly medical, such as a social problem. Furthermore, GPs have a range of community-based resources available that may be more helpful to the patient in coping with the problem.

Box 2.2 illustrates a useful mnemonic highlighting the kinds of responses the GP might make. A definitive diagnosis is not always possible, especially in general practice. However, the patient must always be offered some sort of management of the problem – which may involve a symptomatic remedy (see Chapter 7) or include further investigation or referral for a diagnosis to be achieved. The option of prescribing drugs is dealt with in Chapter 7 and the option of referral to specialists is in Chapter 8.

Reassurance
Many new problems presenting to the GP will be of a minor self-limiting nature. The appropriate action will often be to

---

Box 2.2   **RAPRIOP**

RAPRIOP is a mnemonic to highlight the available range of responses to a patient's problem:

- R   Reassure
- A   Advise
- P   Prescribe
- R   Refer
- I   Investigate
- O   Observe
- P   Prevent

reassure the patient that the problem is not a serious one – reassurance is often talked of as if it were equivalent to a medicine. We will say things like, 'I reassured him it was nothing to worry about' or 'I gave him a lot of reassurance'. Reassurance is not a medicine dispensed according to need by a benevolent doctor, rather, it is a mental process that occurs (or fails to occur) in the mind of a patient. Whether or not reassurance results from a consultation depends on:

- the information the doctor provides the patient about the complaint
- how well this information is targeted at the source of the patient's worry
- how trustworthy the patient judges this information to be.

The information provided must be presented in an easily comprehended manner. Avoid the use of jargon and keep the message simple. Important messages may need to be repeated. To target reassurance to the source of the patient's worry the doctor needs to discover what that worry is. This is not simply a matter of asking the patient what it is (although this may be sufficient sometimes). Patients may be reluctant to admit to their worries, fearing that to admit them may make them look foolish – it may require some subtlety of approach to ascertain the source of the worry. However, if it is correctly identified, then the message can be targeted towards addressing it. The trustworthiness of the information will depend on the patient's attitudes to trusting doctors in general and on the relationship they have with the doctor giving the information. These issues are further discussed in Chapter 9.

While reassurance must not be given too early in the diagnostic process (as it may subsequently prove inappropriate if the patient has a serious health problem), neither should it be withheld unnecessarily while a precise diagnosis is pursued. If arriving at a precise diagnosis may take some time the patient should be reassured that the problem is being taken seriously and the diagnosis will be pursued. If serious possibilities have been ruled out, even though a diagnosis has not yet been arrived at, it may be reassuring to the patient to know this. Even if a serious diagnosis is in the process of being explored it may also reassure the patient to know this rather than be told nothing at all. False reassurance, for example telling the patient there is nothing seriously wrong and not to worry when a serious diagnosis is being contemplated, must be avoided. It damages trust in the doctor–patient relationship when the patient eventually learns that the reassurance was misleading. Once lost, trust is difficult to restore yet it remains critical to effective ongoing care.

Complete reassurance is never possible because all diagnosis is on a probabilistic not a certainty basis (especially so in general practice). It is not necessarily desirable either as a completely reassured patient might not come back on another occasion if similar symptoms develop. Reassurance, therefore, is not so much about removing or relieving patients' anxieties but rather about helping patients set anxiety levels appropriate to the threat to their health.

Advising patients

Closely allied to reassurance is the concept of advising patients. Box 2.3 lists some areas were GPs may be called upon to offer advice.

Patients seek advice from their GP on personal and social problems as well as medical. Doctors need to be particularly cautious in these areas as they are no more qualified than the patient to decide on the best course of action. For such

---

Box 2.3 **Types of advice GPs may be called upon to offer**

- Prevention of health problems and protection of health
- Diet
- Exercise
- Other advice re lifestyle, e.g. smoking cessation
- Home remedies and other self-care
- Over-the-counter treatments
- How and when to take medicines
- When to stop taking medicines
- How to spot adverse reactions of medicines
- Personal/social problems

non-medical areas it is generally best to try and facilitate the patient in making personal decisions and to avoid offering directive advice. This approach is often referred to as 'non-directive counselling'.

Even when advising on problems clearly in the GP's area of competence it is still best not to be too directive. Seek the patient's opinion with regard to the feasibility of implementing any advice offered and be prepared to discuss compromise proposals because, ultimately, the patient is the final arbiter of what to do. By adopting a more collaborative approach it is more likely that the agreed plan of action will be followed than if the doctor simply gives orders the patient does not agree with (see also Chapter 7 on non-compliance and Chapter 9 on doctor–patient communication).

Investigating the patient's problem

Tests are used in general practice to:

- make diagnoses
  - ruling out diseases (in general practice these are usually unlikely but potentially serious conditions)
  - ruling in diseases (not usually necessary for mild or self-limiting illnesses but essential for serious or chronic conditions)
- monitor the progress of disease
- monitor for the potential side effects of medicines
- screen asymptomatic patients for indicators of early disease
- reassure the patient or carers that a disease has been ruled out.

The range of investigations available to GPs varies considerably from place to place but is generally increasing over time (Table 2.3). In many places GPs have full access to virtually every blood test that is routinely available anywhere else in the health service. The range of radiological investigations available varies rather more, though in most places GPs have access to most or all forms of plain X-ray and ultrasonography. GPs also have increasing access to more specialised forms of radiological investigation such as CT scanning but they rarely have direct access to any form of

Table 2.3
Commonly used tests in general practice

Type of test	Type of specimen	Common examples
Haematology	Venous blood	FBC
		Serum ferritin
		Vitamin B12
		Folic acid
		ESR
Biochemistry	Venous blood	Urea & electrolytes (Na, K)
		Liver function tests (albumin, bilirubin, AST, ALT, γGT)
		Renal function tests (creatinine, uric acid)
		Thyroid function tests (T3, T4, TSH)
		Blood glucose
		HbA1c
		Cardiac enzymes (CKMB and T, AST, LDH, aldolase)
Serology/ immunology	Venous blood	Rheumatoid factor
		Anti-nuclear antibodies
		Anti-mitochondrial antibodies
		Anti-DNA antibodies
		Specific antigens (hepatitis titres, Helicobacter titre, ASOT etc.)
		RAST test
Serology	Urine	Pregnancy test (hCG)
Bacteriology	Urine	Midstream specimen of urine (MSSU)
Bacteriology	Swabs	Throat swab
		Wound swab
		High vaginal swab
		Chlamydia swab (special transport medium)
Radiology	X-rays	Chest X-ray
		Plain film of abdomen (PFA)
		X-ray of bones and joints
Radiology	Ultrasound	Obstetric
		Abdominal
		Pelvic
		Renal

invasive radiological investigation. Physiological investigations – such as lung function studies, electro-physiological studies etc. – still tend to be restricted to specialist access.

Whatever investigations GPs have access to it is important they are used responsibly – to do otherwise is both wasteful and potentially dangerous (especially if the investigation is invasive or involves radiation). Only undertake investigations where there is clearly a likelihood that the potential benefits of the investigations outweigh the potential risks, where the results of the investigation will have a direct bearing on decisions about the management of the patient's problem and where there is a reasonable chance of some benefit to the patient. The doctor should know enough about the test to be able to address these issues.

Observation

Given the non-serious and self-limiting nature of many problems presented to GPs it is important that they do not intervene too actively, posing the patient risks of unnecessary investigations or treatments or incurring the health service the costs of inappropriate referrals. However, observing the patient, sometimes referred to as 'masterly inactivity', is not a simple matter. It is important to allow for the possibility that your judgement that the problem is benign and self-limiting is wrong by ensuring that the patient will be reviewed if the problem develops in unanticipated ways. This is called 'safety netting' (see Chapter 4).

Observation can also refer to the monitoring of patients with long-term health problems. In this regard, it is important to know what needs to be monitored, how often it needs to be checked and what the doctor's response to changes in the parameters being monitored should be. It is also important that the patient understands that such observation is ongoing (and, indeed, should be encouraged to self-observe) and will come to the doctor at the required intervals or when a change in the condition merits this (see Chapter 5).

Further Reading

Fraser R C 1999 Clinical method: a general practice approach. Butterworth Heinemann, Oxford

McWhinney I R 2004 A textbook of family medicine, 2nd edn. Oxford University Press, Oxford

Sackett D, Haynes R B, Tugwell P, Guyatt G 1991 Clinical epidemiology: a basic science for clinical medicine. Lippincott Williams and Wilkins, New York

Acute emergencies

When a patient presents to a GP with new symptoms there are three important possibilities to consider:

- is it a benign self-limiting illness (the majority of instances in general practice)?
- is it the first presentation of what will turn out to be a long-term health problem?
- is it an acute medical emergency (Box 3.1)?

Acute emergencies are rare in general practice, but GPs must be able to spot them and respond appropriately.

General approach

The general approach to a possible emergency includes the following:

- make a rapid global assessment of the whole situation
  - any ongoing dangers

Box 3.1 Some important medical emergencies that
may present to a general practitioner

- Collapse
- Coma
- Chest pain
- Poisoning
- Shock
- Fits
- Acute severe breathlessness
- The acute abdomen
- Obstetric emergencies
- Deranged/confused patients
- Suicide/threatened suicide
- Road traffic accidents
- Industrial accidents
- Domestic accidents

  - the number of victims
  - the behaviour of the uninjured
  - how help is to be summoned
- make a specific assessment of the condition of any one
  or more patients
  - determine if they are conscious or unconscious
  - breathing or not breathing
  - whether or not a pulse is present
- prioritise according to ATLS (acute trauma and life
  support) criteria i.e. airways, breathing and circulation.

When emergencies occur in the community (as opposed to
hospital) there are some important implications. Generally
speaking:

- less equipment is available
- fewer drugs are available (but ambulances increasingly
  come supplied with equipment and drugs a doctor
  might need)
- general practitioners may lack all the skills for
  managing emergencies (especially in urban practice

where these skills are used less and, hence, tend to atrophy)
- some element of 'crowd control' is often required
- the nature and type of emergency is less predictable and so it is harder to be prepared for all eventualities (lateral thinking and improvised solutions may be required).

The unconscious patient

A patient who is unconscious, not breathing and pulseless is either dead or in cardiorespiratory arrest. If there is any doubt it is generally safer to assume the latter and commence full cardiopulmonary resuscitation (CPR) immediately. This should be performed by people trained in the technique. Check for a pulse and check the airway is unobstructed. If there is no pulse commence external cardiac compressions and mouth-to-mouth resuscitation or Ambubagging in a ratio of 30:2. Further details of this technique are beyond the scope of this book but all medical students should be trained in this vital skill. Health and safety regulations governing workplaces require that there should be people trained in first aid, so the probability of there being someone trained in CPR is quite high in many situations. A doctor, if present, may be able to make a more precise diagnosis, and treatment more specific to the cause may also be provided (see below).

Obviously, if a reasonably precise diagnosis can be made by a doctor present appropriate specific treatment can be given, if available (see details below). Most vital of all is that someone takes charge of managing the overall situation and that every effort is made to keep everyone calm and in control.

Box 3.2 lists some of the more important causes of unconsciousness.

Box 3.2 Important causes of unconsciousness

- Cardiac arrest
- Head injury
- Stroke
- Alcohol intoxication
- Overdose
- Diabetes
  - hypoglycaemia
  - hyperglycaemia
- Subarachanoid haemorrhage
- Epilepsy
- Meningitis/encephalitis
- Hypothermia
- Shock – hypovolaemic
- Syncope
- Psychogenic (hysteric)

Box 3.3 Key features of acute myocardial infarction

- Crushing central chest pain
- Breathlessness
- Nausea (with or without vomiting)
- Sensation of 'impending doom'
- Visible distress
- Pale and sweating

Some commoner medical emergencies

Acute myocardial infarction (AMI)

See Box 3.3 for the key features. Atypical presentations – such as a feeling of indigestion – are not uncommon and what appears to be a typical picture may represent something other than myocardial infarction, such as a severe angina attack or pulmonary embolism. Definitive diagnosis will require an electrocardiograph (ECG) and a determination of cardiac enzyme levels. However, if there is enough evidence to suggest that myocardial infarction is even reasonably likely, the situation should be treated as for acute myocardial infarction until such time as a more definitive diagnosis can be made. ECG is also useful for the detection of cardiac arrhythmias that are a common and dangerous complication of AMI. Many GPs now carry ECG machines.

In a case of suspected AMI the following steps need to be taken:

- Call an ambulance – be sure to mention that it is suspected AMI as a cardiac ambulance (if available) will have specially trained emergency medical technicians (EMTs), ECG and defibrillation equipment, and thrombolytic therapy on board.
- Administer parenteral analgesia – opiates are preferred but the risk of inducing vomiting means that they are usually given with an anti-emetic (a combination of morphine and the anti-emetic cyclizine).
- Give aspirin – usually as a chewable form. Aspirin is an anti-platelet agent that has been proven to reduce the risks of further infarction – the earlier given the better.
- Administer oxygen if available.
- Sublingual nitrate should also be given.
- Monitor pulse and blood pressure.

Early administration of a thrombolytic, e.g. streptokinase, to suitable patients is also a high priority. The shorter the interval between the onset of myocardial ischaemia and administration of a thrombolytic (called 'pain to needle time') the less myocardium is likely to be lost to infarction and the better the prognosis for the patient – 90 minutes is the target. Thrombolysis is usually carried out in hospital, although in remote areas it may be undertaken by an appropriately trained and equipped GP (see also 'Chest pain' p. 64).

Acute shock

See Box 3.4 for the key features of shock. Shock is a much-used word in the lay media that often refers to people's psychological state after a traumatic event, but it has a more specific medical meaning that refers to a physiological state

Box 3.4 **Key features of shock**

- Pallor
- Clamminess
- Weak pulse
- Altered consciousness

characterised by low blood pressure and decreased perfusion of all body tissues. Two major types of shock are recognised:

- hypovolaemic shock is typically associated with the loss of large quantities of blood
- cardiogenic shock is associated with an acute disruption of cardiac function (such as AMI, see above).

The essentials of emergency management are:

- administer oxygen
- elevate the legs above the level of the heart
- administer intravenous fluids if the cause is thought to be hypovolaemia.

Immediate hospital admission is, of course, obligatory.

Acute severe dyspnoea

Box 3.5 lists some of the possible causes of acute severe dyspnoea. Details on how to differentiate between these causes and how to manage them is beyond the scope of this book and may be found in textbooks of medicine (see Further Reading).

Left ventricular failure (pulmonary oedema)

Box 3.6 lists the key features of left ventricular failure (LVF). Acute LVF may occur in the context of a myocardial infarction, though it can also occur in patients with a variety of other cardiac conditions. It is important to try and determine a cause. General management regardless of cause includes:

- treatment with oxygen (30–60%) – commenced immediately

Box 3.5 Some causes of acute severe dyspnoea

- Acute asthma attack
- Pulmonary embolus
- Pneumothorax
- Pulmonary oedema (LVF)
- Pneumonia
- Adult respiratory distress syndrome
- Chronic obstructive pulmonary disease (COPD)
- Laryngeal obstruction
- Pleural effusion
- Cardiac tamponade

Box 3.6 Key features of left ventricular failure

- Breathlessness (dyspnoea) especially on exertion or on reclining (e.g. paroxysmal nocturnal dyspnoea)
- Tachycardia possibly with gallop rhythm
- Weak pulse
- Crackles at both lung bases (although in severe cases the crackles can be quite widespread)

- a loop diuretic e.g. furosemide – given intravenously, if possible
- intravenous morphine – calms the patient and reduces sympathetic overdrive.

Nitrates, e.g. sublingual glycerine trinitrate, may be useful for vasodilatation but should **not** be given if the patient is hypotensive. An ECG will often identify the cause. Immediate transfer to hospital is required for further management and monitoring.

Acute asthma attack

Box 3.7 lists the key features of acute asthma (asthma attack). The mainstay of management is nebulised beta-agonist such as salbutamol accompanied by intravenous or oral corticosteroids as appropriate to the urgency and severity of the

Box 3.7   Key features of acute asthma

- Severe dyspnoea
- Intense respiratory distress
- Tachypnoea
- Cough and/or wheeze, or possibly 'silent chest' if very severe
- Inability to talk for any length of time
- Use of accessory muscles of respiration
- Subcostal recession (especially in children)
- Tachycardia
- Pallor or possibly central cyanosis

situation. Oxygen (60%) should also be administered if available. If peak flow returns to within 10% of normal for that patient immediately after nebulisation and there were no ominous features the patient might be followed up in general practice. If the attack is severe or the response to nebulisation is poor the patient must be transferred to hospital immediately. A silent chest is a very ominous feature, indicating a need for immediate ventilation.

Acute abdominal pain

Acute abdominal pain is a reasonably common presentation in general practice with myriad possible causes, details of which may be found in textbooks of surgery. For the general practitioner the issue is which patients can be safely managed in the community and which should be referred to hospital (Boxes 3.8 and 3.9).

In women of childbearing age complications of pregnancy, such as ectopic pregnancy, need to be considered too. Pregnancy also limits the range of possible treatments for other causes of acute abdominal pain.

Abdominal pain, where serious causes can be excluded, may be treated with simple analgesics e.g. paracetamol. Non-steroidal anti-inflammatories are best avoided because of the risk of adverse gastric effects.

Any patient with new onset of acute abdominal pain should be kept under close review as many serious causes

Box 3.8 Indications for admission of patients with acute abdominal pain

- Patients in severe pain
- Patients in whom a surgical treatment is likely to be required (e.g. suspected appendicitis, acute perforation)
- Patients with major constitutional upset such as low blood pressure, rapid pulse or respiration
- Patients with a rigid abdomen, rebound tenderness or absent bowel sounds
- The very young and the very old
- Patients in whom a confident diagnosis cannot be made

Box 3.9 Patients with acute abdominal pain who might be managed in the community

- Mild to moderate abdominal pain without other gastrointestinal symptoms or signs
- Where a clear diagnosis can be made with reasonable confidence
- Where the patient is not at risk from other diseases or age or lack of social supports, to allow management at home
- Acute gastroenteritis without dehydration
- Lower urinary tract infection (cystitis)
- Renal colic if diagnosis established, there is no pyrexia and the patient responds to analgesics administered by the GP
- Cholecystitis if diagnosis has been established and there is no pyrexia or jaundice
- Diverticulitis if diagnosis has been established and there is no pyrexia

43

of acute abdominal pain do not fully manifest themselves at the outset of symptoms.

Acute confusion

Box 3.10 lists some of the commoner causes of acute confusion or confusional states that might present in general practice. Every effort should be made to identify and treat the cause of confusion. Meanwhile, there are a few guidelines

> **Box 3.10   Common causes of acute confusion that may present in general practice**
>
> - Infection
> - Drugs/alcohol
> - Stroke
> - Psychosis
> - Shock/subarachnoid haemorrhage
> - Severe pain of any cause e.g. acute retention
> - Epilepsy
> - Various metabolic and endocrine diseases, especially diabetes

for the management of all confused patients regardless of the cause of the confusion:

- Talk calmly and move slowly, avoiding any movement or posture that might be seen as threatening.
- Try and ensure that people not involved in helping the patient are kept well away.
- If there is someone known to the patient their help should generally be sought, unless the patient is threatening them due to, say, a paranoid delusion.
- Try to reassure the patient that they are not in danger of any harm and that you are trying to help them.
- Pharmacological sedation should only be a tactic of last resort.

There may be a risk of violence – this needs to be assessed but care should also be taken not to assume or overestimate this. Containing and dealing with the violent patient is a specialised area and requires special skills and training beyond the scope of this book.

Poisoning

- Try to identify the poison or poisons. In cases of deliberate overdose it is very common for people to have ingested more than one poison and/or to have taken alcohol with whatever else they may have taken.

Box 3.11 **Telephone numbers of poisons centres**
- **UK:** 0870 6006266 (the call will be directed to the relevant local poisons information centre)
- **Ireland:** 01 837 9964 or 01 809 2568 (for the national poisons centre)

- Try to assess the quantity consumed – though one should err on the side of overestimating rather than underestimating this.
- Try to determine whether the poisoning was accidental or deliberate. In deliberate self-poisoning there may be indicators such as a 'suicide note'.
- Manage the poisoning itself *and* any underlying mental health problem.
- Assess the state of consciousness. An attempt to rouse the patient, if not awake or alert, should help determine this. If the patient is deeply unconscious life support procedures (see above) may be required.
- Trying to induce emesis is not always appropriate and should only be done where there are no risks associated with vomiting the poison up again and where the patient is sufficiently alert and cooperative to avoid risk of inhalation. Activated charcoal is more likely to be useful and less likely to be harmful but is not always readily available in community settings. The further management of cases of poisoning is a specialised area and should be undertaken in hospital unless the GP is very confident that the nature and quantity of the poison taken do not constitute a danger. Further guidance should be sought from regional poisons centres (Box 3.11).

Identifying risk of suicide

A very important task in general practice is to try and identify and deal with potential suicides. A patient who is considering suicide may consult a doctor but will only occasionally declare this. This is a very difficult emergency situation where the urgent nature of the patient's problem may not be immediately obvious. The key is to always be alert to the possibility. While the majority of suicides are committed by people with existing mental health problems, a significant minority do not have such an antecedent history. Furthermore, it is also said that up to half the patients presenting to GPs who are clinically depressed are not diagnosed as such by the GP. Patients with depression often present, at least initially, with physical complaints.

Assessing a patient's suicidal risk involves asking some fairly explicit questions about suicidal ideation. It used to be thought that asking people about suicidal thoughts would prompt them into such action but this is now known not to be the case. Indeed, it may be that, by being allowed to air their problems to a caring professional, the risks of completing the act may be reduced somewhat. This does not mean the questions have to be blunt such as asking if patients have thought of 'topping' themselves – a graduated approach is advised (Box 3.12).

The more concrete and active a person's suicidal plans the greater the risk. Generally speaking, active suicidal ideation is an indication for immediate hospital admission – involuntary admission if voluntary admission cannot be negotiated. Milder forms of suicidal thinking can sometimes be managed in the community as long as there is easy access for the patient to emergency follow-up. In such a situation the availability of the means of suicide should be reduced as much as possible – removing knives, medicines etc.

Box 3.12 A graduated approach to assessment of suicidal risk

- Ask first about thoughts about the future
- Progress to asking about any thoughts about self-harm
- Then ask specific questions about any suicidal fantasies or actual plans

Accidents in the home

In the UK approximately 10 000 people die from accidental injury, 4000 of these occurring in the home. It is the leading cause of death in children. It is estimated that there are about 2.8 million accidents in homes in the UK compared with about 300 000 road traffic accidents. The most vulnerable to accidents in the home are children, followed by elderly people (over 65 years) – although half the fatalities occur in adults of working age. The commonest causes of accidents in the home are falls and fires. In children, accidental poisoning and various forms of crushing or cutting injuries, burns and electrocution are also quite common.

A substantial proportion of victims of accidents will attend or be brought to accident and emergency departments. Where a GP is called to an accident in the home the situation will need to be managed according to the nature of the accident, the number of victims (or potential victims) and the nature of injuries probable or apparent. Management of the unconscious patient and acute poisoning are noted above. Mild trauma may be manageable by the GP but in any instance of major trauma or risk of undisclosed trauma, such as fractures or injuries to internal organs, referral to hospital will be required.

In the case of accidents to children GPs also have to bear in mind the possibility of non-accidental injury and follow the appropriate local procedures for dealing with actual or potential non-accidental injury. Domestic violence can also result in apparently accidental injuries to adults as well as children. Abuse of elderly persons by their carers, too, is beginning to be recognised as a problem in society. Thus it is important to take a clear history of any incident of accidental injury. Be alert to inconsistencies in the history or disproportions between injuries received and the alleged cause or other indicators of the possibility that what is presented as an accident is not one.

GPs have an important role in the reduction of accidents in the home. When visiting patients in their home we can see aspects of the home environment that might present possible risks – loose fitting carpets, trailing electric flexes, unguarded fires etc. As house calls become a less prevalent part of general practice activity such opportunities are reducing – this makes it all the more important that the most is made of what opportunities do arise. When an elderly patient seems to be developing a history of recurrent falls or other mishaps a home visit might be worthwhile. Parents of young children are frequent visitors to GPs' surgeries and some advice on safety in the home may be provided by a proactive GP. Bodies such as the Royal Society for the Prevention of Accidents (RoSPA) publish guidelines on how to prevent accidents in the home.

Management of road traffic accidents

Urban GPs will rarely be called to road traffic accidents but for many rural GPs it is an important part of their work. Any doctor may happen to be first on the scene of an accident and will usually be expected to know what to do. Here are some guidelines:

- Reduce the risk of further accidents by setting up some kind of warning for other traffic.
- If possible, get any injured people off the road, though only if it is safe to move them (see below).
- Make a global assessment of the accident scene. How many vehicles are involved and how many potential casualties are there? Be aware of the possibility of unexpected casualties such as pedestrians or cyclists caught up in what might initially appear to be a car-only accident or of casualties flung out of cars and ending up some distance from the crash site.
- Try and prioritise casualties. Remember that the most seriously injured often make the least noise.
- Summon help as early as possible, giving as much information as possible to assist emergency services correctly identify the location. On dual carriageways and motorways you should specify the direction of

travel of the lane in which the accident has occurred.
Give the numbers of casualties and some estimate of
their injuries.
- Do not try and move people who might have neck
injuries or, indeed, who may have major bone fractures
unless a real risk of fire makes this imperative.
- Remain calm and try to exert reasonable control on the
behaviour of others at the scene.

Other types of accident

Other types of accident are managed according to similar
principles:

- Manage the entire accident scene and not just the
casualties. The risk of further accidents or exacerbating
the dangers is a common feature of accident scenes and
is a constant trap for the unwary or inexperienced.
- Take care to avoid becoming a casualty, e.g. from
electrocution in electrical accidents or being
contaminated in toxic spills etc.
- Summon appropriate help as soon as possible. Police
and ambulance are usually both required to manage
the scene as well as the injured. When summoning
help, the more information about location, type of
accident, number and nature of casualties and so
on that can be given the better. If specialist help is
required the emergency services will usually summon
this.
- Casualties should be dealt with in priority order
according to the severity of their injuries and threat to
life, as long as this is consistent with containing
self-danger.

Accidents in the community, in common with all emergencies, are inherently unpredictable. Training in first aid
and accident management is very valuable and should be
part of the training of all doctors but you will also need to
be flexible and resourceful to deal with the unanticipated
aspects that are a feature of most emergencies.

Acute and self-limiting illness

52

Introduction

Illnesses generally present with symptoms. In chronic illnesses (see Chapter 5) the symptoms are usually recurrent and predictable from the nature of the illness. However, for patients presenting with new symptoms the first task of the GP is often to determine whether the symptoms are possibly indicative of a serious disease, or of a more benign, self-limiting disease, or whether they might even be due to normal physiological responses. For example, palpitations can be caused by anxiety, heart disease or benign tachycardia due to physical exertion. Most symptoms presenting to GPs are indicative of benign self-limiting illness but the task of the GP is to sort these from the rarer potentially more serious causes.

The steps to dealing with acute self-limiting illness in general practice are:

- determining that the disease is, indeed, benign and likely to be self-limiting
- considering why the patient has chosen to consult
- explaining the benign and self-limiting nature of the condition to the patient
- agreeing a management plan (which will often be implemented by the patient alone)
- 'safety netting' i.e. establishing a review process whereby the patient will be reviewed if the problem develops in ways that suggest it is more serious than first supposed (see Chapter 2).

53

Generalised symptoms

Fever (pyrexia)

Defined as an oral temperature over 37.3°C, fever is typically associated with infectious illnesses, the majority of which in general practice are of viral origin (Box 4.1). Certain illnesses are associated with particular patterns of fever (e.g. quatrain fever associated with malaria) but such fever patterns are rare in general practice. Fever persisting for more than 3 weeks without remission or a cause being identified is considered 'pyrexia of unknown origin' (PUO) and would usually be referred to hospital for investigation.

Box 4.1 Causes of pyrexia

Likely	**Possible**
Influenza	Travel-acquired infection
Upper respiratory tract	e.g. malaria
infection	Chronic pyelonephritis
Other simple viral	Tuberculosis
infections e.g. with	Carcinoma
corona viruses/	Lymphoma/leukaemia
Coxsackie virus	Rheumatoid arthritis
Epstein–Barr virus	Zoonoses
infection (glandular	Cytomegalovirus infection
fever)	Hepatobiliary infection
Enteroviral infection	HIV/AIDS
Abscess	Infective endocarditis
Pelvic inflammatory	Drug-induced, e.g.
disease	allopurinol,
	antihistamines,
	cephalosporins,
	cimetidine, quinidine,
	phenytoin,
	sulphonamides
	Lyme disease

Diagnostic pointers

Specific symptoms in one bodily system often give a pointer to the cause of a fever, e.g. cough and fever point to the respiratory system. Lifestyle, occupation, hobbies or recent activities placing the patient at risk of exposure often provide pointers too, e.g. recent foreign travel points to increased likelihood of exotic infections, work with animals increases likelihood of zoonoses etc. Weight loss often accompanies chronic infection but may also be a pointer to malignant disease (see below). Itching may be associated with hepatobiliary disease and with leukaemia and lymphoma. Night sweating is associated with lymphoma and with tuberculosis. A history of valvular cardiac disease and/or a cardiac murmur is suggestive of infective endocarditis.

Management

The underlying cause of the fever, if it can be identified, should be managed appropriately. For the fever itself anti-pyretic medicines (particularly paracetamol) are appropriate and increased fluid intake is necessary to counteract the risk of dehydration secondary to the pyrexia. Particularly in children, tepid sponging is also a useful means of effecting rapid temperature reduction. This is best achieved by covering the child in tepid water and allowing the water to evaporate off, i.e. the child should not be dried. The water must be tepid (i.e. close to normal body temperature) for this treatment to be effective. Cold water causes peripheral vaso-constriction and may prevent dissipation of the raised body temperature through evaporation. Rapid application of effective anti-pyretic measures is particularly important in children under 5 who are prone to febrile convulsions.

Tiredness (fatigue)

See Box 4.2 for likely and possible causes of fatigue.

Diagnostic pointers

A description of the patient's typical day may reveal a pattern likely to lead to stress and/or overwork. Enquiry about sleep pattern may, likewise, point to life stressors but may also give indications of the likelihood of depression. Other more specific indicators of depression may be detected by enquiry after mood, view of the future etc. Anaemia, if severe, may be associated with chest pain or palpitations but will more often be associated with general pallor. Enquiry about common sources of blood loss (e.g. menorrhagia in women, gastrointestinal symptoms in either sex) may also provide useful pointers. Recent viral infection may be revealed by a general review of recent health as may thyroid disease and diabetes – although these latter two may also produce more specific symptoms (for details consult a general medicine text). Tiredness accompanied by weight loss is much more likely to have a sinister origin and a more thorough search for the cause is merited in this scenario.

Box 4.2   Causes of fatigue or unexplained tiredness

Likely
Stress/overwork
Insomnia
Depression
Anaemia
Recent viral illness
Hypothyroidism
Diabetes mellitus

Possible
Infective mononucleosis
    (glandular fever)
Chronic fatigue syndrome
Organ failure (heart,
    kidney, liver)
Hyperthyroidism
Alcoholism
Drug misuse
Adverse reaction to
    medications (e.g.
    beta-blockers)
Malignancy
Chronic infection (e.g. TB,
    UTI)
Connective tissue disease
    (RA, SLE etc.)
Chronic neurological
    disease
Other endocrine disease
    (e.g. Addison's disease)

Management

Where tiredness appears to be a product of the patient's lifestyle, change in lifestyle may be advised but patients will generally have to make their own decisions regarding how much they can change. Paradoxically, increasing exercise levels can help reduce feelings of tiredness and lethargy where these are lifestyle related. The management of insomnia and of depression is dealt with below. The diagnosis of anaemia can only be made on the basis of a determination of haemoglobin level and the treatment should be directed towards the underlying cause (see general texts for further details).

The management of tiredness related to endocrine disease should likewise be related to the specific disease (see general texts). Given the large number of possible causes of tiredness investigation with a battery of blood tests including full blood count, biochemical profile, thyroid function tests and so on is a commonly used strategy – but a thorough history, and especially a comprehensive systems review, will often provide more systematic pointers that may allow the search for a cause to be narrowed.

Weight loss

Box 4.3 lists the likely and the possible causes of unexplained weight loss.

Diagnostic pointers

Weight loss in older people is always potentially sinister and must be fully investigated until a cause can be found. Investigations will initially be targeted on any system with associated symptoms but they should also include a detailed dietary history as in some old people weight loss may be due to poor diet. In children, too, weight loss is potentially serious although it is sometimes more feared than real – it might be worth taking several consecutive readings before initiating invasive investigations. A good history of social conditions, parenting techniques and nutritional practices may also reveal the cause of potential failure to thrive.

Some people with hectic lifestyles eat too infrequently and too little, with resultant weight loss. Weight loss is

Box 4.3 Causes of unexplained weight loss

Likely	Possible
Lifestyle-related	Diabetes mellitus
Depression	Eating disorder
Hyperthyroidism	Malignancy
	Chronic infection (e.g. TB)
	HIV/AIDS
	Alcoholism
	Drug misuse
	Major organ failure (heart, liver, kidney)
	Inflammatory bowel disease
	Coeliac disease
	Malabsorption syndromes
	Malnutrition

also a common accompaniment to 'stress', possibly due to an effect on appetite. Depression will be accompanied by features of low mood, sleep disturbance etc. Hyperthyroidism may be indicated by heat intolerance, excessive sweating, palpitations and, possibly, exophthalmos (if due to Graves' disease).

Diabetes presenting with weight loss would usually be insulin-dependent diabetes and so would be accompanied by thirst, polyuria, polydipsia and polyphagia. In eating disorders weight loss may not be complained of by the patient but is apparent to others. In young women amenorrhoea is another possible indicator, as are acid dental erosion (due to repeated self-induced vomiting) and electrolyte imbalances (due to vomiting and/or laxative abuse). The patient will often think they are over- rather than underweight and the problem may be a recurrent one. Sorting out the myriad causes of weight loss can be quite difficult and might require successive rounds of history taking, examination and investigations before the cause is finally discovered. The more underweight the patient and the more rapid the weight loss the stronger is the case for early referral to a specialist.

Management

The management of weight loss comprises a good balanced diet with a level of calorie intake appropriate to the patient's age, gender, reproductive status (pregnant and lactating women need higher calorie intake), occupation, activity levels etc. If a specific cause is identified for the weight loss, then appropriate management of this problem is required.

Weight gain

Box 4.4 gives the likely and less likely (but still possible) causes of weight gain.

Diagnostic pointers

Most people who put on weight do so because of an imbalance between their calorie intake and their energy expendi-

Box 4.4 Causes of weight gain

Likely	**Possible**
Simple obesity	Iatrogenic (steroids, oestrogen, sulphonylureas)
Pregnancy	
Hypothyroidism	
Heart failure	Depression (with comfort eating)
Nephrotic syndrome	
Alcoholism	Polycystic ovarian disease
	Acromegaly
	Cushing's disease
	Other endocrine disorders
	Congenital disorders e.g. Prader–Willi syndrome

ture. Most pregnant women present because of a missed period but sometimes, especially if the possibility of pregnancy has not occurred to them, weight gain may be the presenting feature. Patients with hypothyroidism will usually have other features of hypothyroidism such as cold intolerance, hoarseness, constipation etc. but these can be subtle because of the gradual onset of this condition. Weight gain due to oedema can occur as a result of either heart failure or renal failure and will show features typical of dependent oedema, including gravitational distribution and pitting on pressure. Other features of these conditions will usually be present. Less common causes of weight gain have other specific features that will be revealed by appropriate investigations.

Management

Helping patients to lose weight is a major challenge. Keys to success included adopting a supportive, non-judgemental attitude; promoting realistic goals; combining calorie intake reduction with increased physical activity; involving significant others in the patient's weight loss efforts; regular follow-up with weighing at each review; and rewarding patient's successes with praise. The stages-of-change model (see Chapter 6) is also applicable. There are two pharmacological treatments to help with weight loss, orlistat and sibu-tramine. These are mainly indicated in patients with morbid obesity (BMI greater than $30 \, \text{kg/m}^2$) and/or patients with complications of obesity such as diabetes mellitus. Details of their use are beyond the scope of this book.

Chest symptoms

Cough

See Box 4.5.

Diagnostic pointers

Weight loss and chronic cough suggests either carcinoma or tuberculosis – haemoptysis makes these diagnoses even more likely. Haemoptysis accompanied by pleuritic chest pain and/or respiratory distress strongly suggests possible pulmonary embolism. Rhinorrhoea, pyrexia, and sore throat in the absence of lower respiratory tract symptoms such as chest pain, tightness, wheeze or haemoptysis is probably just a simple cold or upper respiratory tract infection (URTI).

Box 4.5 Causes of cough

Likely	Possible
Upper respiratory tract infection	Chronic airways disease including COPD and bronchiectasis
Lower respiratory tract infection, particularly pneumonia	Tuberculosis
	Sarcoid
Asthma	Fibrotic lung disease
Smoker's cough	Foreign body
	Cystic fibrosis
	Lung cancer
	Other respiratory tract cancer
	Pulmonary embolism
	Cardiac failure

Lower respiratory tract infections (LRTIs) are more likely in the very young, the very old, smokers, patients with pre-existing respiratory disease or immunocompromised patients. They may be preceded by URTI symptoms. The presence of pyrexia and production of sputum do not, per se, distinguish between URTI and LRTI, although greater severity and/or persistence of these symptoms may be pointers to an increased likelihood of LRTI. Raised respiratory rate and other signs of respiratory distress also make LRTI more likely. Chest signs, i.e. rhonchi or crepitations, are possibly indicative of bronchitis and pneumonia respectively. Wheeze is the quintessential sign of asthma. Other pointers to asthma include history of atopy, history of allergy in general, exercise-induced symptoms, recurrent symptoms and nocturnal symptoms (especially cough). Cough may be the main or only symptom of asthma (especially in children). A good response to bronchodilator medication is also a useful diagnostic indicator of likely asthma. A peak flow >10% below expected is strongly suggestive of asthma, although the true test of asthma is being able to show that this reduction in peak flow is reversible.

Cough is usually chronic in a patient who has smoked quite heavily (20 cigarettes per day or more) for several years and may also occur in people exposed to high levels of environmental tobacco smoke. Other causes of persistent cough may only be revealed after extensive investigation and/or specialist referral.

Management

Symptomatic self-management with fluids, anti-pyretics and steam inhalations are the mainstays of treatment of URTIs. It is important to avoid unnecessary antibiotics because of risks of fuelling antibiotic resistance in the community and because of risks of medicalising the condition. LRTI is more likely to be bacterial (although it may still be viral). An appropriate broad-spectrum antibiotic such as amoxicillin will be sufficient in most cases of community-acquired infection. Chest X-ray (CXR) is not generally needed in the GP setting but may be indicated in older patients and smokers (to rule out cancer). For more details on asthma management see Chapter 5; see Chapter 6 for more details on encouraging smoking cessation.

Wheeze
See Box 4.6.

Diagnostic pointers

Wheeze that comes and goes or is worsened by exercise, cold air or exposure to inhaled allergens and is relieved by bronchodilators is asthma. Wheeze accompanied by pyrexia and a productive cough (especially if sputum is yellow or green) is more likely to be due to acute bronchitis. This is more likely in a smoker and is particularly likely in someone who has a chronic productive cough or is known to have chronic obstructive pulmonary disease (COPD). Wheezing due to left ventricular failure – what used to be called 'cardiac asthma' – will usually be accompanied by other indicators of cardiac disease such as a history of myocardial infarction. The wheeze is mainly inspiratory (as opposed to expiratory in typical asthma) and may be succeeded by a cough, producing pink frothy sputum. Basal crackles are also indicative of left ventricular failure. Carcinoma of the bronchus, commoner in older than in younger people, may be associated with weight loss, persistence of infective signs in spite of adequate antibiotic therapy and possibly haemoptysis. Inhaled foreign bodies are more common in small children and may be associated with unilateral chest signs (obstruc-

Box 4.6   Causes of wheeze

Likely	**Possible**
Asthma	Inhaled foreign body
Acute bronchitis	Carcinoma of the bronchus
Left ventricular failure (cardiac asthma)	

tion of the trachea being quite unusual) including either rhonchi and/or possibly signs of atelectasis distal to the foreign body.

Management

The management of asthma, chronic bronchitis/COPD and cardiac failure is covered in Chapter 5. The management of carcinoma of the bronchus and inhaled foreign bodies is beyond the scope of this book.

Breathlessness/difficulty breathing (dyspnoea)
See Box 4.7.

Diagnostic pointers

For pointers to URTI and distinguishing URTI from LRTI see 'cough' above. For pointers to asthma and cardiac causes see 'wheeze' above. Hyperventilation typically occurs in someone prone to anxiety (particularly panic attacks) and will resolve rapidly if the patient re-breathes from a *paper* bag. Pulmonary embolism is typically associated with severe chest pain and haemoptysis in addition to breathlessness. Pleural effusion may be a sign of cardiac, renal or liver failure or a complication of lung cancer or tuberculosis. It is associated with findings of dullness to percussion over part or all of one or more lung fields and may also be associated

Box 4.7 Causes of difficulty in breathing

Likely	**Possible**
Upper respiratory tract infection	Pulmonary embolism
Acute bronchitis	Pleural effusion
Pneumonia	Diabetic ketoacidosis
Asthma	Carcinoma of the bronchus with lobular collapse
Left ventricular failure	Pneumothorax
Hyperventilation	Aspiration pneumonitis

with signs and/or symptoms of a preceding DVT (deep vein thrombosis).

Diabetic ketoacidosis is a complication of diabetes and may occasionally be the initial presentation of this diagnosis. It will usually be preceded by a typical history of symptoms of diabetes or it may rapidly progress to unconsciousness. Carcinoma of the bronchus with lobar collapse may be indicated by typical features of carcinoma such as weight loss and anaemia, as well as features of chest examination of atelectasis (collapse) including diminished air entry, area of reduced resonance and, possibly, crackles. Confusion accompanying breathlessness may indicate hypoxia, sepsis or metabolic abnormalities (such as ketoacidosis) and requires urgent hospital admission.

Management

Dyspnoea accompanied by hypoxia is treated with oxygen. Where there is a pleural effusion symptoms will usually be relieved if the effusion is drained. Treatment of dyspnoea is otherwise directed to treatment of the underlying cause.

64

Chest pain

See Box 4.8. See also 'Acute myocardial infarction' p. 38.

Diagnostic pointers

The key diagnosis not to be missed in a patient presenting with chest pain is acute myocardial infarction (AMI). The older the patient, the more severe the pain, the longer the duration of the pain (particularly if greater than 30 minutes), the more the pain is associated with other symptoms (particularly cardiorespiratory symptoms and symptoms of haemodynamic shock), the more likely the pain is to be due to AMI. Pain of AMI also has a crushing quality and is generally localised to the centre of the chest, but often radiates to the left shoulder, arm or jaw and may have been precipitated by exertion or emotion. It is difficult to distinguish from the pain of angina although it is typically more severe and may be recognised by the patient as more intrin-

Box 4.8 Causes of chest pain

Likely	Possible
Anxiety	Pleurisy
Costochondritis (Tietze's syndrome)	Pneumothorax
Angina	Peptic ulcer, especially with perforation
Acute myocardial infarction	Shingles
Reflux oesophagitis	Mastitis
Chest trauma	Bornholm disease
Muscle strain	Cardiomyopathy
	Aortic aneurysm

sically frightening. In a patient not known to have ischaemic heart disease the distinction may be immaterial in a general practice setting as all such patients will be managed as if they have had an AMI and will be sent to hospital by cardiac ambulance (if possible) until the diagnosis can be established. In a patient already known to have ischaemic heart disease and/or a history of angina the distinction can still be difficult to make but short duration of symptoms and relief achieved by rest or administration of a nitrate are more indicative of an anginal attack.

Another reasonably common diagnosis that may be associated with severe retrosternal pain and a shocked appearance with pallor and clamminess is spasm of the oesophagus. Pointers to this diagnosis are prior symptoms of heartburn or other upper gastrointestinal disease. While anxiety is a typical accompaniment of AMI, chest pain due to anxiety without AMI is typically associated with an absence of symptoms or signs of shock and more general features of anxiety such as a tendency to worry over a great variety of things, difficulty sleeping, feelings of being hot and sweaty (rather than cold and sweaty). Anxiety about possible cardiac disease is common but such patients will usually have milder, less acute symptoms with few, if any, physical signs.

Chest pain due to musculoskeletal disease will often be associated with some precipitating trauma and will be worse on certain movements and associated with well-localised tenderness on palpation.

Chest pain due to pneumothorax, pleurisy or pulmonary embolism will typically be associated with inspiration and, possibly, relieved by expiration. There may also be other respiratory symptoms such as dyspnoea, cough (possibly with haemoptysis) and chest signs such as wheezes or crackles. However, it should be noted that AMI associated with left ventricular failure will also produce respiratory symptoms and signs, especially dyspnoea and basal crepitations.

Management

The management of AMI or suspected AMI is covered in Chapter 3. General management of ischaemic heart disease is covered in Chapter 5. The management of other conditions is dictated by their location and nature. The presentation of a patient with chest pain in the absence of any likelihood of serious underlying pathology provides a good opportunity for promotion of cardiovascular health including screening for hypertension, hypercholesterolaemia, checking smoking history and other possible modifiable risks of cardiovascular disease (see also Chapter 6 – prevention). Patients with chest pain will often be concerned or have become concerned about their risk of cardiovascular disease – this anxiety also needs to be managed. Usually this is achieved by simply explaining the features of the case that make AMI a very unlikely diagnosis. Sometimes more specific anxiety management may need to be undertaken.

Palpitations

See Box 4.9 for causes.

Diagnostic pointers

Anxiety will often be apparent from the patient's general demeanour and apparent in the way the patient speaks. ECG will usually identify the precise cardiac arrhythmia unless it is intermittent (as atrial fibrillation can be).

Box 4.9   *Causes of palpitations*

Likely	**Possible**
Anxiety	Hyperthyroidism
Sinus tachycardia (due to	Menopause
exercise, fever, stress)	Prescribed medicines (e.g.
Cardiac arrhythmia	digoxin, nifedipine)
Drugs and alcohol (esp.	
nicotine and caffeine)	

Tachycardia can have many causes, most of them, in a general practice setting, quite benign. Excess alcohol and/or caffeine are two worth considering. Hyperthyroidism, although often associated with a tachycardia, will only occasionally present with palpitations. Menopause usually need only be considered in women of the relevant age.

Management

- anxiety (see below)
- tachycardia (manage according to cause)
- cardiac arrhythmia (refer to more detailed medicine texts).

ENT symptoms

Sore throat
See Box 4.10.

Diagnostic pointers

Acute sore throat is more likely to be viral if symptoms are rapid in onset, of short duration and associated with temperature and cough. Enlarged tonsils and/or pus on the tonsils do not make bacterial pharyngitis or streptococcal tonsillitis any more likely. A unilateral swelling behind a tonsil makes the diagnosis of peritonsillar abscess or quinsy more likely. Infective mononucleosis is ruled out in the

Box 4.10   Causes of a sore throat

Likely	**Possible**
Acute viral infection e.g. rhinovirus	Quinsy (peritonsillar abscess)
Acute streptococcal infection (Lancefield B)	Infective mononucleosis
	Haematological malignancy (leukaemia)
	Agranulocytosis or aplastic anaemias
	Carcinoma of throat
	Diphtheria

absence of a membrane on the palate/tonsils, but is more likely if there are palatial petechiae or generalised lymphadenopathy, especially splenomegaly.

Haematological malignancy is of low, but roughly equal, likelihood in most age groups and should be considered in any patient who seems more generally unwell than would be expected or who fails to recover as expected. A similar picture may indicate agranulocytosis or aplastic anaemia but in the latter case drug-induced causes should be an active consideration. Diphtheria is exceedingly unlikely in developed countries especially if the patient has been immunised (as would be normal in such countries).

Management

There is clinical trial evidence to support the view that non-steroidal anti-inflammatories are helpful for the symptoms of sore throat. A commonly recommended route for anti-inflammatory medication is in the form of aspirin gargles. Other strategies believed to help include consumption of extra fluids and rest (including extra bed rest). Prevention should also be raised and there is good reason to suppose that smokers who give up smoking are less likely to suffer further episodes of pharyngitis. Although commonly prescribed for sore throat, partly on the basis that 30% of episodes can be related to an infection with *Streptococcus pyogenes*, antibiotics are not generally indicated or recommended. In populations with low incidence of streptococcal infection complications, such as rheumatic heart disease and acute glomerulonephritis, the research evidence does not support routine use of antibiotics for sore throat or even streptococcal sore throat.

Antibiotics are also thought to reduce the risk of suppurative complications such as quinsy – although the evidence to support this is also weak and such risks need to be traded off against the risk of adverse effects of antibiotics, which are reasonably common. While antibiotics should generally be avoided, a compromise may be reached with many patients whereby they are given a prescription for an antibiotic, which is only to be used if symptoms do not abate. Studies have shown that such a strategy will reduce antibiotic prescribing while avoiding patients feeling their symptoms have not been taken sufficiently seriously.

Runny nose/nasal obstruction
See Box 4.11.

Box 4.11   Causes of a runny or stuffy nose

Likely	**Possible**
Common cold	Septal deviation
Hay fever	Nasal polyps
Perennial (allergic) rhinitis	Enlarged turbinates (often accompanies chronic allergic rhinitis)
Vasomotor rhinitis	Nasal trauma, including fracture and haematoma
	Foreign body (especially small children)
	Iatrogenic (e.g. doxazosin)
	Cancer of nose, nasal passages including sinuses

Diagnostic pointers

- *Common cold.* Acute onset associated with pyrexia and often sore throat and sneezing. More common in spring and autumn and may be associated with contact with other sufferers.
- *Hay fever.* Occurs particularly in spring and summer and sufferers are usually affected at the same time each year. Worse when pollen count is high and if exposed to high pollen levels. Associated with sore, runny, itchy red eyes and possibly with throat and/or chest symptoms (wheeze etc.).
- *Perennial rhinitis.* Symptoms persist throughout most or all of year. Associated with diminished smell and/or taste.

Management

- *Common cold* – see cough.
- *Hay fever.* Avoid allergens if possible. Steroid nasal sprays – especially if nasal symptoms predominate. Sodium cromoglycate eye drops can be helpful when eye symptoms predominate. Many patients will require oral anti-histamines of which the non-sedating varieties are generally more popular. All these treatments are available over the counter but may also be prescribed.
- *Perennial rhinitis.* Occasionally an allergen or allergens can be identified by careful history taking, especially of the waxing and waning of symptoms. House dust mite is a common culprit and measures to reduce house dust mite can be helpful. Nasal steroids are the mainstay of treatment.

Nosebleeds
See Box 4.12.

Diagnostic pointers

- *Spontaneous.* More common in children. May be associated with allergic or perennial rhinitis or even

Box 4.12   Causes of nosebleeds

Likely	**Possible**
Spontaneous (although often associated with nose-picking and/or sneezing)	Foreign body (especially small children)
	Drugs e.g. anticoagulants
	Hypertension
Nasal infection with ulceration	Excess use of nasal sprays e.g. steroids
Allergic rhinitis	Liver disease
	Cancers
	Trauma esp. unhealed fracture
	Coagulopathies e.g. haemophilia
	Hereditary haemorrhagic telangiectasia

acute coryza. Often recurrent but bleeding usually easily controlled.

- *Nasal infection.* Associated with soreness in the nose and possibly with malodorous purulent discharge (though these are also associated with foreign bodies in the nose). Ulceration may be apparent on examination with nasal speculum.
- *Allergic rhinitis* – see above.

Management

First aid for nosebleeds consists of getting the patient to sit down and lean forward over a bowl. Then press the nose just below the end of the nasal bone for 10 minutes or until the bleeding has stopped. Cautery of Little's area can be helpful for recurrent nosebleeds, especially if this area is hyperaemic. Nasal infections, if limited and not associated with any area of surrounding erythema, may be treated with antibiotic ointment such as Bactroban (mupirocin) or Naseptin (neomycin and chlorhexidine). For treatment of allergic rhinitis, see above – nasal obstruction.

Hoarseness

See Box 4.13.

Diagnostic pointers

- *Acute laryngitis.* Often associated with other features of upper respiratory tract infection e.g. runny nose, sore throat, fever. Acute onset and short duration are typical.
- *Hypothyroidism.* Associated with other features of hypothyroidism such as weight gain, cold intolerance, skin thickening etc.
- *Singer's nodules.* Benign tumours more common in people such as singers who use their voice a lot in intensive ways. Singer's nodules will usually be visualised on indirect laryngoscopy.
- *Carcinoma of the larynx.* Unlikely in younger people and is particularly associated with pipe smoking. Other indicators of cancer such as anaemia and weight loss make this diagnosis more likely.
- *Oesophageal reflux* will be associated with other GI symptoms, particularly heartburn.

Management

Patients complaining of hoarseness regardless of cause need to be told to rest their voice by trying not to speak any more

Box 4.13 Causes of hoarseness

Likely	Possible
Acute laryngitis (usually viral)	Singer's nodules
Overuse of voice	Carcinoma of the larynx
Hypothyroidism	Oesophageal reflux
Smoking	Acute epiglottis
	Post intubation
	Recurrent laryngeal nerve palsy
	Hysterical aphonia

than strictly necessary and to avoid shouting or straining of the voice in particular. Smokers should be encouraged to quit. Hoarseness persisting for more than 6 weeks should usually be referred to an ENT surgeon.

Gastrointestinal symptoms

Indigestion/dyspepsia

Dyspepsia is a medical term that has been coined to encompass a range of sometimes rather vague symptoms complained of by patients. The symptoms include vague feelings of discomfort (as opposed to pain), nausea, heartburn and feelings of abdominal distension or fullness – all of which tend to centre on the epigastric area. The closest lay term to encompass these sensations is probably indigestion. See Box 4.14 for the causes.

Diagnostic pointers

Acute gastritis is suggested by sudden acute onset and may be associated with a recent history of over-indulgence, especially in alcohol. Gastro-oesophageal reflux disorder is suggested by a history of reflux, i.e. sensations of stomach contents or 'water brash' coming up the oesophagus, and is also more likely if the patient is overweight. Peptic ulcer disease is associated with more severe symptoms akin to

Box 4.14   Causes of dyspepsia

Likely	Possible
Acute gastritis	Cholelithiasis
Gastro-oesophageal reflux disorder (GORD)	Gastric cancer
	Oesophageal cancer
Hiatus hernia	Liver disease
Peptic ulcer disease	Pancreatic disease
Non-ulcer dyspepsia	Ischaemic heart disease
	Irritable bowel syndrome

actual pain and pain which is relieved by food and aggravated by abstinence from food. Smoking also makes peptic
ulcer disease more likely though not smoking does not rule
it out. Non-ulcer dyspepsia is associated with dyspepsia for
which other causes cannot be found, and as such, does not
really have features that rule it in. It is ruled out when other
diagnoses are made.

Cholelithiasis is more usually associated with abdominal
pain than dyspepsia and may be associated with jaundice
if the bile duct becomes blocked. Gastric or oesophageal
cancer will be associated with weight loss and, possibly,
anaemia. Oesophageal cancer is more likely to be associated
with partial or complete dysphagia. Liver disease may be
associated with jaundice, or less dramatically with hypo-
proteinaemia and/or raised liver enzymes on routine blood
tests. Pancreatic disease may be associated with pain, too,
and may also be associated with jaundice. Vomiting is a
prominent feature of pancreatitis – the pain may be relieved
by leaning forward.

Management

Simple dyspepsia (especially if short term and infrequent)
can be treated with antacids. More frequent or longer episodes of dyspepsia, as well as making investigation more
necessary, may also respond more effectively to H_2 blockers.
Peptic ulcer disease needs investigation for the presence of
Helicobacter pylori and, if present, this will need treatment
with 'triple therapy'. For currently recommended regimens
for the treatment of *H. pylori* see the British National
Formulary. Gastro-oesophageal reflux disorder may respond
to antacids, ideally with alginates, but more persistent
symptoms may justify prescribing of a proton pump inhibitor (see also Chapter 5). Gastrointestinal cancers will need
specialist investigation and treatment.

Heartburn

This is a retrosternal burning sensation associated with
regurgitation of acidic stomach contents into the lower end
of the oesophagus. See Box 4.15 for its causes.

Box 4.15   Causes of heartburn

Likely	**Possible**
Gastro-oesophageal reflux	Carcinoma of the oesophagus
Acute gastritis	Scleroderma
	Drugs affecting oesophageal motility e.g. theophylline, calcium channel blockers
	Angina pectoris
	Pregnancy

Diagnostic pointers

Gastro-oesophageal reflux is associated with unhealthy dietary practices including eating late in the evening and eating large quantities of fatty and/or spicy foods, and with consumption of alcohol. Obesity is also a common accompaniment. Hiatus hernia may be detected on gastroscopy or barium swallow.

Acute gastritis is also associated with dietary indiscretion and alcohol consumption but is, typically, more acute and short lived. Carcinoma of the oesophagus is the biggest fear in a patient presenting with heartburn. It is more likely in older patients, in patients who smoke and particularly if they have other symptoms of cancer such as weight loss or anaemia.

Angina pectoris can present with symptoms very similar to those of reflux oesophagitis but there may be other indicators of cardiac ischaemia such as exacerbation by exertion or emotion. Heartburn is a common complaint during pregnancy but is usually more pronounced in the third trimester and so is not a usual symptom for pregnancy to present with.

Management

Although proton pump inhibitors are very effective in relieving heartburn regardless of its cause, the effect only lasts for as long as the drugs are taken. Furthermore, for many patients a simple antacid or perhaps H_2 antagonist (which are generally cheaper than proton pump inhibitors) will suffice. More importantly, patients with oesophageal reflux should be informed about the dietary and lifestyle contributions to their condition and encouraged to try and minimise or eliminate their symptoms by lifestyle adjustments and without the need for medicines. Weight reduction is important where obesity is a contributing factor and avoiding stooping or bending will also help where there is incompetence of the gastro-oesophageal sphincter.

Acute abdominal pain

See Box 4.16 for causes (see also Chapter 3, 'Abdominal pain' p. 42).

Diagnostic pointers

The acute abdomen can be diagnostically very taxing. Appendicitis, in particular, is important not to miss because

Box 4.16 Causes of acute abdominal pain

Likely	**Possible**
Gastroenteritis	Irritable bowel syndrome
Acute gastritis	Diverticulitis (especially in the elderly)
Peptic ulcer	Pancreatitis
Cholelithiasis (gallstones)	Pyelonephritis
Appendicitis	Muscle strain of abdominal wall muscle
	Perforation – stomach, duodenum or bowel
	Ulcerative colitis
	Crohn's disease
	Intestinal obstruction (e.g. due to carcinoma of the bowel)
	Hepatitis
	Dissecting aortic aneurysm
	Ketoacidosis
	Depression

timely surgical intervention is very effective and perforation of an appendix is potentially fatal. For the GP, therefore, if there is any possibility of appendicitis the patient should be referred to hospital – a precise diagnosis is neither necessary nor often possible in general practice. However, more often in practice there will be pointers to more likely specific causes.

Abdominal pain associated with a short history of vomiting and/or diarrhoea (especially in the context of a recent outbreak of gastroenteritis or possible food poisoning or recent foreign travel) may be acute gastroenteritis. A preceding history of dyspepsia (see above) or of pain relieved by food and worse at night may indicate a peptic ulcer.

Pain localised to the right hypochondrium, especially if radiating to the right shoulder and exacerbated by fatty foods, may indicate cholelithiasis and associated biliary colic. If a patient with these features is pyrexial in addition and has a positive Murphy's sign they may have cholecystitis.

Appendicitis classically begins with pain in the umbilical area, which subsequently moves to the right iliac fossa and is associated with anorexia, pyrexia, tachycardia, nausea and vomiting. However, not all of these symptoms will be present in every case. Abdominal examination may reveal rebound tenderness in the right iliac fossa but a retrocaecal appendix may only induce tenderness on rectal examination. It is for this reason that a rectal examination may be necessary if the GP wants to rule out retrocaecal appendicitis. However, if the decision has already been made to admit the patient to hospital is it not necessary (and is not usually desirable) for the GP to carry out this examination (see Chapter 3 regarding which patients need to be admitted).

Any form of intra-abdominal perforation and pancreatitis will typically present with a patient who is quite obviously ill, often possibly with signs of shock (pallor, sweaty, tachycardia and low blood pressure) and abdominal examination may reveal either localised rebound tenderness or, if peritonitis is more established or extensive, board-like rigidity. Older patients with a history of constipation and or rectal bleeding may be suffering from carcinoma of the colon or, more commonly, diverticulitis.

Management

The management of abdominal pain should be directed primarily towards the cause of the pain. However, where benign causes are probable and there is no risk of missing an important diagnosis such as appendicitis, simple analgesics may be appropriate. Non-steroidal anti-inflammatories (NSAIDs) are usually best avoided in the treatment of abdominal pain because of the risk they might exacerbate peptic ulceration that might be the underlying cause of the pain.

Nausea and vomiting

Virtually all of the conditions that can give rise to vomiting can also cause nausea without vomiting, hence the two symptoms are considered together here. Furthermore, while nausea and vomiting tend to be thought of as specifically gastrointestinal symptoms, they can occur in a great many other conditions – particularly in vestibular disease and neurological conditions (such as migraine and brain tumour) – and can be induced by virtually all known drugs in at least some patients. Note, also, that in children vomiting is a common accompaniment of pyrexia and may be due to virtually any illness than can raise a child's temperature (see Box 4.17).

Diagnostic pointers

Because of the great many conditions in most bodily systems that can give rise to nausea and vomiting, the investigation of the cause should be focused, initially, on whatever system appears to have related symptoms. Thus nausea or vomiting with abdominal pain points to possible gastrointestinal causes; headache or other neurological symptoms points to possible neurological disease and so on. A thorough drug history including self-medication is also very important given the propensity of a great many drugs to cause nausea/

Box 4.17 Causes of nausea and vomiting

Likely	Possible
Peptic ulcer disease	Labyrinthitis
Acute gastritis	Ménière's disease
Gastroenteritis	Diabetes – hypo and
Irritable bowel disease	hyperglycaemic states
Migraine	Raised intracranial
Pregnancy	pressure e.g. tumours or
Urinary tract infection	intracranial haemorrhage
Drugs e.g. antibiotics,	(any type)
cytotoxics,	Meningitis
theophyllines, digoxin	All causes of acute
Anxiety (nausea probably	abdominal pain (see Box
more commonly induced	4.16) can cause
by anxiety than actual	nausea/vomiting
vomiting)	Constipation
	Inflammatory bowel
	disease
	Hepatitis
	Depression
	Renal failure
	Glaucoma
	Acute myocardial infarction
	Various cancers especially
	of the gastrointestinal
	tract
	Bulimia nervosa

vomiting. The presence of a fever leads one to look for sources of infection. A menstrual history may disclose a period of amenorrhoea and point to pregnancy as a possible cause. While anxiety frequently causes nausea one needs to take care to rule out physical causes before concluding that nausea or vomiting are due to anxiety alone.

Management

The management of nausea and vomiting is directed towards the cause, if this can be discovered. While anti-emetics can be effective in relieving symptoms of nausea or vomiting, care should be taken to establish the cause of the symptoms before opting for such symptomatic remedies. In benign self-limiting causes of nausea and vomiting such as gastroenteritis the use of anti-emetics is probably unnecessary as the condition will usually settle quite quickly without treatment and the risks of adverse effects (such as dystonia) possibly outweigh any benefits for many patients. When nausea/vomiting are thought to be drug-induced a risk–benefit judgement decision will also have to be made regarding whether or not to stop the putatively offending drug or continue with it (possibly in combination with an anti-emetic). Remember, also, that profuse or prolonged vomiting can lead to dehydration (especially in children and others prone to dehydration) so ensuring adequate fluid intake is an essential part of the management of vomiting.

Diarrhoea
See Box 4.18.

Diagnostic pointers

Infective gastroenteritis is ruled in by its rapid onset and relatively short course. There may be an identifiable source, such as possibly contaminated food. A slight fever is also indicative of a possible infective cause. Inflammatory bowel disease, such as ulcerative colitis or Crohn's disease, is more likely where there is blood and/or mucus in the stool, although this can also be a feature of some more severe types of infection such as dysentery.

Box 4.18 Causes of diarrhoea

Likely	**Possible**
Viral gastroenteritis	Ulcerative colitis
Bacterial gastroenteritis	Diverticulitis
Recent antibiotics	Food intolerance
Dietary indiscretion	(hypersensitivity)
Traveller's diarrhoea	Antibiotic/drug-induced
	Irritable bowel syndrome
	Bowel cancer

Systemic features such as anaemia or weight loss are also more indicative of serious causes such as inflammatory bowel disease or, possibly, malignancy. Diverticulitis is characteristically associated with older people and would be suggested by the presence of pain, raised temperature and possibly nausea and vomiting. Food intolerance would be more common in younger patients and children and might be associated with other atopic conditions such as eczema and asthma.

Management

The main risk in diarrhoea is that of dehydration and so the mainstay of therapy is fluid replacement. There is a variety of over-the-counter remedies, and some available on prescription too, but none of these is recommended for the routine treatment of acute diarrhoeal illness. Although many episodes of diarrhoea are associated with bacterial gastroenteritis this does not mean antibiotics are good for the condition. Indeed, because of their propensity to alter normal bowel flora and their relative lack of effectiveness, antibiotics are not generally recommended except for some particular organisms (once these have been identified).

An important preventive measure is to insist on thorough hygiene, especially of hands. Patients with diarrhoea (especially if due to gastroenteritis) may also need to notify employers or desist from food preparation within their work to reduce the risk of spreading the infection. Good hygiene, care in the preparation of food and consumption of food within use-by dates are important elements of prevention that should be instituted.

Constipation
See Box 4.19.

Diagnostic pointers

Enquiry about the patient's diet may give indications of this being a causative factor. A diet low in roughage, erratic meal times, and rushed meals associated with an irregular

Box 4.19 Causes of constipation

Likely	**Possible**
Poor diet	Inflammatory bowel
Immobility	disease (i.e. ulcerative
Irritable bowel syndrome	colitis or Crohn's
	disease)
	Hirschsprung's in children
	Intussusception in children
	Bowel obstruction
	Carcinoma of bowel
	Diverticulitis

lifestyle are all factors likely to contribute to what is effectively a physiological form of constipation. Similarly, a lack
of mobility, particularly if recent or recently worsened, can
be pointers to this as a cause of the constipation. Remember
that the immobility itself may not be complained of but one
may still be able to adduce immobility as a likely factor
where this is a history of joint pain or other conditions likely
to be immobilising the patient.

Irritable bowel would be indicated by a more chronic
picture, other gastrointestinal symptoms and, possibly,
associated psychological features. Abdominal pain is a
common accompanying feature and may not be particularly
helpful in sorting the diagnoses – although if it is severe it
may be indicative of a more serious cause.

Nausea, and particularly vomiting, are definitely more
ominous features and may be indicative of more serious
causes such as bowel obstruction. Unfortunately, from a
diagnostic point of view, their absence does not preclude
more sinister causes. Constitutional features such as a raised
pulse or temperature are more unequivocally sinister
features and may suggest causes such as diverticulitis or
inflammatory bowel disease.

More chronic constitutional features such as weight loss
or signs of anaemia are even more clearly ominous and
should prompt a rigorous search for a serious cause such as
carcinoma or inflammatory bowel disease.

Management

Given that the commonest cause of constipation is poor diet, the mainstay of treatment is also dietary. In particular, to relieve constipation an increase in the proportion of fibre in the diet is generally needed. Relative dehydration can also contribute to constipation and so adequate fluid consumption of fluids without diuretic properties (i.e. not tea, coffee or alcoholic beverages) needs to be maintained. Having ruled out serious causes and where dietary measures fail, or where the patient requires a quicker result, one might recommend laxatives – many of which are available over the counter. However, laxatives are best avoided in children and long-term use can lead to hypokalaemia and atonic bowel.

Abdominal distension/abdominal mass
See Box 4.20.

Diagnostic pointers

What is perceived as abdominal distension noted by an otherwise seemingly well patient is often simple obesity.

Box 4.20 Causes of abdominal distension/mass

Likely
Obesity (not strictly
    distension but often
    mistaken for it)
Constipation
Pregnancy
Fibroids
Irritable bowel syndrome

Possible
Intestinal obstruction
Carcinoma of stomach,
    pancreas, bowel, liver,
    uterus or ovary
Hepatomegaly (see
    medicine texts for
    causes of hepatomegaly)
Splenomegaly
Ascites
Aortic aneurysm
Urinary obstruction
Polycystic disease of the
    kidney
Hydronephrosis
Nephrotic syndrome

Lack of or infrequent bowel movements may lead one to think of constipation. Amenorrhoea will make one think of possible pregnancy. Associated pain, weight loss, vomiting or fever are all ominous features and should lead to a thorough search for a more specific cause and/or specialist referral. Abdominal examination should locate the distension to one or more affected organs if the condition is organ-specific. Careful examination should also detect distension due to ascites.

Management

Management should be related to the specific cause which, given the number of potentially serious causes, should be determined before any treatment is instituted.

Rectal bleeding

See Box 4.21

Diagnostic pointers

Painless bleeding after a bowel movement is most likely due to a haemorrhoid. Pain with bleeding on defecation is more likely to be related to anal fissure, while pain with bleeding not related to defecation might be a thrombosed external haemorrhoid. A pilonidal sinus will be apparent on exami-

---

Box 4.21 Causes of rectal bleeding

Likely	Possible
Haemorrhoids	Ulcerative colitis
Anal fissure	Colorectal cancer (benign
Pilonidal sinus	or malignant)
Diverticular disease	Trauma
(especially in elderly)	Intussusception (children
Gastroenteritis/dysentery	only)
	Meckel's diverticulum
	(children only)
	Anti-coagulants
	Coagulopathy

nation of the perianal area. Diverticular disease is more common in the elderly and will be associated with more generalised abdominal pain, fever and a history of constipation.

More severe forms of gastroenteritis may be associated with blood in the stools but vomiting and diarrhoea are usually more prominent features and there may be a history of a risk of consumption of contaminated food and/or foreign travel. In ulcerative colitis there may be mucus and blood in the stool. Symptoms may be intermittent and chronic although initial presentation in a fairly toxic state is another possible presentation that would lead to immediate referral to a specialist.

Colorectal cancer is more common in older patients and may be associated with altered bowel habit, weight loss and anaemia. There may be a family history. Any patient over 50 with a history of rectal bleeding should be investigated for possible colorectal cancer.

Management

There are a variety of proprietary haemorrhoid creams, ointments and suppositories available – both on prescription and over the counter – with a variety of components designed to relieve symptoms of pain and itching and reduce bleeding. More important, though, is the need to reduce straining at stool (the commonest cause of haemorrhoids), which will usually require a high-fibre diet and possibly the use of a stool softener or bulking agent. Surgical treatment may be required where these measures do not work and this may involve either sclerosant injections or rubber banding. Anal fissures are also related to constipation and straining at stool and measures to reduce these problems are part of the management. Many of the proprietary haemorrhoid preparations may be useful for anal fissures too, although other preparations containing local anaesthetics are also used. Occasionally surgery may be required.

Pilonidal sinuses may need to be incised and drained but complete excision of the sinus is necessary to avoid recurrent infection. For treatment of gastroenteritis see Diarrhoea (above).

Genitourinary symptoms

Urinary frequency
See Box 4.22.

Diagnostic pointers

Frequency with dysuria is a urinary tract infection more often than not but, if recurrent, and no infection can be proven bacteriologically, it may be classed as 'urethral syndrome'. Asking about consumption of substances with known diuretic properties such as xanthines (found in tea and coffee) or alcohol may identify the cause of urinary frequency in the absence of pain. Otherwise one may have to check for the more serious and rarer causes such as diabetes and cardiac failure. Pregnancy may be revealed by a history of amenorrhoea and/or a positive pregnancy test.

Management

Simple lower urinary tract infections (UTIs) are quite common in young sexually active women and are usually treated with an appropriate antibiotic – guided by known

---

Box 4.22   Causes of urinary frequency

Likely	Possible
Lower urinary tract infection (cystitis)	Upper urinary tract infection (pyelonephritis)
Urethral syndrome	Diabetes mellitus
Excessive diuretic substances (incl. tea, coffee and alcohol)	Cardiac failure
	Psychogenic polydipsia
Early pregnancy	Diabetes insipidus

local sensitivity patterns. Antibiotics with known potential for tetragenicity should be avoided if there is any risk of the woman being pregnant. Women with urethral syndrome or recurrent infections need to be advised about reducing the risk of vagino-urethral transfer of organisms by measures such as appropriate genital hygiene, micturition before and after coitus and the use of lubricants for coitus.

Dysuria

See Box 4.23.

Diagnostic pointers

Dysuria accompanied by frequency is almost invariably due to urinary tract infection or urethral syndrome. If accompanied by vaginal discharge it may be due to a vaginal infection and, in the case of men, a urethral discharge may be indicative of non-specific urethritis or other sexually transmitted infection. Similar symptoms also occur in Reiter's syndrome but other indicators of connective tissue disease (dry eye symptoms and seronegative arthritis) are usually present too.

More chronic dysuria symptoms in an older male may be indicative of prostatitis. Dysuria associated with haematuria might be indicative of a urethral calculus.

Management

For the management of UTI see above. Prostatitis will need a longer course of antibiotics than simple UTI. Management

---

Box 4.23   Causes of dysuria

Likely	**Possible**
Urinary tract infection (esp. lower UTI)	Urethral calculus
Urethritis	Reiter's syndrome
Vaginitis	
Prostatitis	

of vaginal infections is dealt with below (under vaginal discharge). Reiter's syndrome is treated with rest and non-steroidal anti-inflammatories.

Vaginal discharge
See Box 4.24.

Diagnostic pointers

- *Physiological discharge.* A certain amount of vaginal discharge is physiological and it is also normal for the amount and character of the discharge to vary throughout the hormonal cycle and throughout a woman's reproductive life. In the absence of any specific characteristics of the discharge (see below), the absence of any accompanying symptoms and a discharge that peaks in amount mid-cycle, a physiological discharge can often be assumed (at least until appropriate microbiological testing has been completed).
- *Bacterial vaginosis.* A thin, pasty, grey malodorous discharge may indicate bacterial vaginosis.
- *Vaginal thrush.* Candidiasis is associated with a whitish discharge, sometimes described as like cream cheese.

88

Box 4.24   Causes of vaginal discharge

Likely	Possible
Physiological discharge	Dermatitis
Bacterial vaginosis	Herpes simplex
Vaginal thrush (Candidiasis)	Foreign body (e.g. lost tampon or others in children)
Trichomonas vaginitis	
Gonorrhoea	
Chlamydial infection	Discharging Bartholin's cyst/abscess
Atrophic vaginitis (postmenopausal women)	Cervical ectropion
	Cervical cancer
	Vulvovaginal cancer

Itching is a common accompanying feature. Vaginal thrush may be precipitated by use of broad-spectrum antibiotics and use of corticosteroids, and is also more common in patients with diabetes.

- *Trichomonas vaginitis.* Trichomonas is associated with copious, thin, frothy discharge, which is either grey or greenish-yellow in colour. The discharge of trichomonas is said to have a fishy smell.
- *Gonorrhoea.* The discharge associated with gonorrhoea is typically thick and purulent (yellow/greenish) looking.
- *Chlamydial infection.* The discharge associated with Chlamydia is whitish-yellow in colour and relatively odourless but it may only be clearly apparent on speculum examination when it will, typically, be seen to be oozing from the cervical os.
- *Atrophic vaginitis* (post-menopausal women). Atrophic vaginitis occurs in peri-menopausal and post-menopausal women and is associated with itching, burning and soreness. The discharge is usually not that profuse but may be blood stained.

89

Management

If there is a likelihood of sexually transmitted infection the patient should be fully investigated for all forms of STI, including serological tests for syphilis and HIV; all patient contacts should also be traced, tested and treated. This may be more effectively done through a genitourinary medicine clinic if one is readily available. Bacterial vaginosis and tri-chomonas are usually treated with metronidazole. Candida is usually treated with a local preparation (cream or pessary) of an appropriate anti-fungal (clotrimazole or miconazole), both of which are available over the counter and on pre-scription. Recurrent candida may need to be treated with an oral anti-fungal such as fluconazole or itraconazole. The treatment of sexually transmitted infection should be guided by the policies of the local genitourinary medicine clinic.

Amenorrhoea

Amenorrhoea is usually divided into primary and second-ary amenorrhoea. Primary amenorrhoea is the absence of periods in a patient who has never had a period and is very rare in general practice. Secondary amenorrhoea, being more common, is the type dealt with here. See Box 4.25.

Diagnostic pointers

Amenorrhoea in a sexually active woman of reproductive years is most often due to pregnancy. If a pregnancy test is negative enquiry into lifestyle – work, exercise, diet etc. – will often disclose possible stress, weight loss or excessive exercise as possible causes. Polycystic ovary disease may be associated with features of masculinisation (e.g. hir-sutism), acne and obesity. Anorexia and bulimia can be difficult to detect unless they are thought of but anorexia will often become apparent if the woman is weighed in underclothes only. Other causes will be revealed if thorough endocrinological investigations are undertaken but these would only be embarked on if other more likely causes were ruled out.

Management

Management needs to be specific to the cause of the amenorrhoea.

Box 4.25   Causes of amenorrhoea

Likely	Possible
Pregnancy	Anorexia/bulimia
Stress	Hypothyroidism
Weight loss	Hyperthyroidism
Menopause	Prolactinoma
Intensive exercise	Addison's disease
Polycystic ovary disease	Sheehan's syndrome
	Simmond's disease
	(primary pituitary failure)

Musculoskeletal symptoms

Backache
See Box 4.26.

Diagnostic pointers

A patient who walks into the GP's surgery and has no obvious limp or sign of being in great distress is unlikely to have an acute serious condition such as prolapsed intervertebral disc. A history of recent trauma or pain coming on when bending or lifting will most usually be indicative of an acute sprain/strain of the back. Neurological symptoms such as weakness or paraesthesia may be indicative of a prolapsed disc if accompanied by the expected neurological signs of diminished or absent reflexes or diminutions of power or sensation. However, in the absence of confirmatory signs neurological features may be merely indicative of inflammatory swelling around nerves emanating from the spinal cord and hence may be features of a more straightforward strain.

Osteoarthritis is associated more with older patients and is much more likely where there are signs or symptoms of osteoarthritis in other limbs or joints. Likewise osteoporotic vertebral collapse is much more likely where there is already known to be osteoporosis – although vertebral collapse, not

Box 4.26 *Causes of backache*

Likely	**Possible**
Sprain or strain of back	Prolapsed vertebral disc
Sciatica	Osteoporotic vertebral collapse
Osteoarthritis (spondylosis)	
Multiple myeloma	Bony secondaries in malignant disease (esp. cancer of bronchus, breast, prostate and thyroid)
	Psychogenic

infrequently, is the first manifestation of osteoporosis. Thus, osteoporosis needs to be suspected in all older people but particularly in women – and especially if they are post-menopausal and not on hormone replacement or other treatment to prevent osteoporosis.

Metastatic bone disease is obviously more likely in patients already known to have cancer, but it should be suspected in all older patients, especially where there may be other indicators of malignant disease such as weight loss or anaemia.

Management

For acute mechanical back strain the main treatment is analgesia. Paracetamol, if given in adequate doses, is often sufficient, although non-steroidal anti-inflammatory analgesics such as ibuprofen are possibly more often prescribed. There is much debate about the role of rest, but evidence is now more strongly in favour of avoiding too much rest and getting back to normal activity as soon as possible.

Backache is often associated with poor posture and/or poor lifting techniques. Advice on these is important in avoiding the risk of an acute episode developing into a chronic pattern of recurrent backache. Physiotherapists, where sufficiently available, are very good at advising and training people on back pain prevention. This preventive activity is sometimes organised on a group basis in a 'back school'.

Where there is a prolapsed disc but without evidence of any neurological impairment rest may be more appropriate and stronger analgesics such as opiates may be required. Where there is neurological impairment a neurosurgical or orthopaedic opinion is desirable and where the neurological impairment suggests a 'cauda equina' lesion urgent referral to neurosurgery is required.

Pain in single joints
See Box 4.27.

Box 4.27   Causes of pain in single joints

Likely	Possible
Trauma (sprain/strain most common)	Septic arthritis
	Fracture
Repetitive strain injury	Dislocation/subluxation
Osteoarthritis	Reiter's disease
Gout/pseudogout	Malignancy
Rheumatoid arthritis	Chondromalacia patellae (knee)
	Osgood–Schlatter's disease (knee esp. in adolescents)
	Avascular necrosis (especially hip)

Diagnostic pointers

History of recent trauma will indicate a probable traumatic cause, while history of relevant repetitive use may indicate repetitive strain type injury. More severe forms of trauma may cause fracture, dislocation or subluxation of the joint or nearby bones. The nature of such bony injuries will usually become apparent on examining the relevant joint, when displacements or discontinuities become apparent. If in doubt, an X-ray will clarify matters. Osteoarthritis is typically a condition of older people and, while it may present with pain in a single joint, enquiry may reveal pain and/or stiffness in more than one joint. Weight-bearing joints and joints that have been subjected to trauma in the past are particularly vulnerable.

Gout, typically, affects the tarso-pharyngeal joint of the big toe but can affect other joints. Gouty tophi may also sometimes be found in gout sufferers. Rheumatoid arthritis, also, usually affects more than one joint and is associated with red, swollen joints, pyrexia and other symptoms related to connective tissue disease. Septic arthritis is associated with a very red and hot joint and generalised pyrexia, and possibly enlarged lymph nodes in the relevant area. Other conditions can be linked to specific joints. See Further Reading for more information.

Management

Acute trauma and short-lived symptoms can usually be managed with simple analgesics such as paracetamol. More persistent problems associated with possible inflammation such as repetitive strain injuries can be treated with non-steroidal anti-inflammatories and, if very persistent and well localised, with steroid injections. Osteoarthritis should also be managed with simple analgesics and physiotherapy. Various forms of heat treatment can be useful, especially if confined to a single or only a few joints. Non-steroidal anti-inflammatories are also used extensively in the treatment of osteoarthritis, although their use is controversial. Further details of the management of osteoarthritis are covered in Chapter 5.

Acute attacks of gout are treated with NSAIDs – traditionally indomethacin but nowadays diclofenac is a more usual treatment. Gout, if associated with raised uric acid level, may be treated long-term with allopurinol. Because of the significance to future joint health and the risk of untreated or inadequately treated septic arthritis patients should be referred to a specialist. Management of rheumatoid arthritis is discussed in Chapter 5. Septic arthritis is treated with appropriate antibiotics. Fractures and dislocations are managed surgically. See Further Reading for the management of other conditions.

Pain in multiple joints
See Box 4.28.

Diagnostic pointers

Osteoarthritis is typically a condition of older people associated with pain and stiffness in weight-bearing joints in particular. Stiffness typically develops as the day progresses and with increased joint use. Joint swelling does occur but it develops later in the disease and the swelling, while often tender, is not usually red or hot to the touch. In the hands osteoarthritis is associated with Heberden's nodes.

Box 4.28   Pain in multiple joints

Likely	**Possible**
Osteoarthritis	Viral polyarthritis
Rheumatoid arthritis	Ankylosing spondylitis
Other connective tissue	Reiter's disease
disorders e.g. SLE,	Enteropathic arthritis
polyarteritis nodosa etc.	Sarcoidosis
Psoriatic arthropathy	Brucellosis
	Malignancy (particularly
	bony secondaries)

   Rheumatoid arthritis can begin at any age and typically presents with red, hot, swollen joints and joint stiffness, which is worse in the morning or after periods of inactivity. Psoriatic arthropathy is associated with psoriasis (see skin diseases, below, for details of treatment).

   Connective tissue disorders present with a great many different symptoms but, typically, symptoms affecting other bodily systems in addition to the joints will occur.

Management

The management of osteoarthritis and rheumatoid arthritis are both covered in Chapter 5. The management of other connective tissue disorders is quite complex and needs to be tailored to the manifestations of the disease in the particular patient. Key components of treatment include non-steroidal anti-inflammatories, corticosteroids and immunosuppressive drugs. Anti-malarials such as hydroxychloroquine may be used in some connective tissue disorders, such as rheumatoid arthritis and SLE, but are not suitable for others, such as psoriatic arthropathy. Sarcoidosis is treated mainly with corticosteroids. Brucellosis is treated with antibiotics, usually tetracycline.

Swollen joint(s)
See Box 4.29.

Box 4.29   Causes of swollen joint(s)

Likely	**Possible**
Sprain	Septic arthritis
Osteoarthritis	Fracture
Rheumatoid arthritis	Charcot's joint
Bursitis	Other arthritides e.g.
Gout	psoriatic, Reiter's etc.
Ankle swelling only:	Ankle swelling only:

- Congestive cardiac failure
- Nephrotic syndrome
- Venous insufficiency
- Pelvic mass

- Anaemia
- Drug reaction (esp. calcium channel blockers and NSAIDs)
- Protein-losing enteropathy

Diagnostic pointers

In a joint sprain there will usually be a history of preceding trauma and accompanying pain. Pain is also a feature of osteoarthritis, rheumatoid arthritis, gout, fracture and other arthritides. In osteoarthritis large weight-bearing joints tend to be affected – especially the knees in the case of swelling. In rheumatoid arthritis small joints of the hands and feet can be affected and there will often be stiffness in joints in the morning.

Bursitis can occur at the site of many different joints but the swelling is peri-articular rather than of the joint itself. Pain and redness are usual but not invariable features of bursitis. Bursitis may be related to overuse type injuries or pressure on the bursa.

Septic arthritis is associated with a lot of redness of the joint and constitutional symptoms such as pyrexia. It is readily apparent when a joint aspirate is purulent. Charcot's joints are joints damaged secondary to undetected trauma due to loss of sensation as a result of neuropathy. The key feature, therefore, is the accompanying neuropathy.

Swollen ankles have additional possible significance over and above that for other joints as they are the site of oedema associated with a variety of other systemic and vascular conditions, particularly congestive cardiac failure (see

Chapter 5). Vascular and cardiac causes are accompanied by other features of these conditions. Renal causes may be accompanied by polyuria. Venous insufficiency may be apparent through other signs such as the presence of varicose veins.

A pelvic mass causing ankle oedema may only be apparent if the abdomen and pelvis are also examined – although a history of gastrointestinal or gynaecological symptoms may also provide pointers. Unilateral ankle oedema is also a warning of possible pelvic mass. Anaemia will also be accompanied by other signs both of anaemia (pallor, lassitude etc.) and, in more severe cases, cardiac compromise (dyspnoea, palpitations, etc.). Drug reactions will be suspected where the relevant drugs have been taken by the patient. A protein-losing enteropathy may be suggested by gastrointestinal features, especially diarrhoea.

Management

Management of osteoarthritis and rheumatoid arthritis are covered in Chapter 5. Management of gout and septic arthritis are covered above. Bursitis may be treated with nonsteroidal anti-inflammatories but may also need aspiration if it persists. Sprains are treated with rest, ice, compression and elevation of the relevant joint if seen immediately after the injury. If more than several hours have elapsed ice is much less likely to be helpful and in the days after injury heat treatment may be more beneficial. Very severe strains may require more sophisticated treatments such as strapping or possibly even immobilisation. Fractures will always require surgical management. Septic arthritis is treated with appropriate antibiotics. For treatment of other causes see Further Reading.

CNS symptoms

Headache
See Box 4.30.

Box 4.30   Causes of headache

Likely	Possible
Tension headache	Intracranial space-occupying lesion i.e. brain tumour, brain abscess etc.
Upper respiratory tract infection particularly sinusitis	Malignant hypertension
Migraine	Analgesic headache
	Brain haemorrhage
	Head trauma
	Meningitis

Diagnostic pointers

Tension headaches are the commonest type of headache. They are often described as a feeling of tightness or a band surrounding the head, although they may also be described as affecting the front, back or top of the head and will usually be bilateral rather than unilateral. They may be associated with feelings of tenseness elsewhere, especially in the neck muscles, and may also be associated with other features of sympathetic overdrive such as sweating, palpitations, fluttery feelings in the stomach etc. Sometimes there may be an obvious cause of anxiety or tension associated with the headache but they are commonly found in the absence of obvious cause.

Headaches associated with upper respiratory tract infections will, naturally, be associated with other features of upper respiratory tract infection such as pyrexia, rhinorrhoea, sore throat, cough and so on. However, the headache may not appear early in the respiratory infection and the acute symptoms of the URTI may have abated by the time the headache occurs, so the patient may not necessarily associate the two. Headaches are a common feature of acute sinusitis, in which case there will be additional features of nasal obstruction and symptoms specific to sinus infection such as facial pain.

Migraine is sometimes difficult to distinguish from tension headache, particularly where the two conditions co-exist in the same patient – as can be the case. However, migraine is more usually unilateral and will often be associated with nausea and/or vomiting and possibly visual disturbances or photophobia. Migraine is a recurring condition that occurs in attacks. Typical attacks may be preceded by an aura, which may consist of various visual or other neurological symptoms. Severe forms of migraine may also be associated with a variety of neurological disturbances following an attack. Migraine is a familial condition and so a positive family history is a common finding. Some migraine sufferers may also be able to relate their headache to particular circumstances and/or dietary consumption.

Intracranial space-occupying lesions, most commonly brain tumours, can be difficult to distinguish from other causes of headache and should be considered where headaches are particularly severe, persistent or are associated with stable neurological disturbances. The occurrence of anything possibly resembling an epileptic fit is, of course, a significant indicator of likely intracranial pathology and so should be sought where headaches are in any way atypical. Weight loss or anaemia are other features that would suggest malignant disease but in such a case the headache is more likely to be due to a brain secondary. Space-occupying lesions would also possibly be associated with signs of raised intracranial pressure such as papilloedema and/or low blood pressure (where there is brain stem pressure).

Malignant hypertension would be associated with high blood pressure but also with papilloedema. In malignant hypertension the headache may also be accompanied by visual disturbances.

Analgesic headache is a condition associated with overuse of analgesics. This is a potentially confusing condition because the patient may have begun with more ordinary causes of headache, such as tension or migraine, but in their attempts to self-manage they may have used analgesics on too long and regular a basis. When they reduce or stop the analgesia the headache gets worse and so they go on taking analgesia, which then maintains the condition. This cause for the headache should become apparent if one takes a careful history of the headaches and the patient's self-management strategies.

Subarachnoid haemorrhage will usually present with a very acute onset of a very, very severe headache though in some cases there is a less severe headache at the onset that later becomes extremely severe. Subdural haemorrhage is often preceded by head trauma and the onset can be quite insidious. There may be associated drowsiness or a feeling of being fuzzy headed.

Meningitis is usually accompanied by other signs and symptoms of meningeal irritation such as nausea, vomiting, photophobia and neck stiffness.

Management

Once it can be determined that the headache is probably due to tension the use of ordinary analgesics such as paracetamol is reasonable, providing one takes care these are not used in too high a dose or for too long because of the danger of analgesic headache (see above). Other ways of reducing tension such as muscle relaxation techniques, yoga, transcendental meditation, massage etc. are also quite reasonable and can be very helpful. Where there is a clear-cut cause of anxiety or psychological stress anything that can be done to reduce this will also help. Analgesics are also very useful in headache related to upper respiratory tract infection including sinusitis. The use of antibiotics and/or decongestants for sinusitis, although still quite popular among patients and some doctors, is not supported by good research evidence and is not generally recommended.

Migraine may respond quite well to adequate doses of ordinary analgesics such as paracetamol if they are given early enough in the attack. Where the headache is accompanied by significant nausea or vomiting a combination of paracetamol and an anti-emetic such as metoclopramide is also known to be beneficial in many patients. However, there are now more specific remedies for migraine that are designed to modulate the serotonin system, which is believed to be important in the causation of migraine. These are generally very efficacious but are quite a lot more expensive than traditional anti-migraine treatments. They may be justified in more severe cases because loss of work and other capacities to patients may be more significant than the cost of the medicines. The diagnosis and management of the more sinister causes of headache are beyond the scope of this book.

Dizziness
See Box 4.31.

Diagnostic pointers

In the assessment of the patient complaining of dizziness it is important to distinguish between so called 'true vertigo' and dizziness. True vertigo is sensation of rotatory movement of either the patient or the environment. Dizziness is a sensation of impending imbalance or falling over. True vertigo implies either vestibular or cerebellar disease. The Romberg manoeuvre is performed by observing the patient standing with feet in parallel and close together. If standing in this position with eyes closed provokes swaying it

Box 4.31   Causes of dizziness

Likely	Possible
Anxiety	Toxic labyrinthitis e.g. due to aminoglycosides
Acute viral labyrinthitis	
Benign positional vertigo	Ménière's disease
Vertebrobasilar insufficiency	Acoustic neuroma
	Multiple sclerosis
Cervical spondylosis	Herpes zoster oticus (Ramsay–Hunt syndrome)
Postural hypotension	
	Stroke
	Cerebellar disease
	Alcohol (either acute inebriation or secondary cerebellar disease)

suggests vestibular disease (or possibly impaired proprioception) whereas if swaying occurs when eyes are both open and closed it is more likely to be cerebellar disease. The co-existence of a positive Romberg's with nystagmus is almost pathognomonic of cerebellar disease.

The Hallpike manoeuvre is a method to provoke vertigo and/or nystagmus by stimulation of the semicircular canals. The patient lies down with the head over the end of the examination couch. The examiner tilts the patient's head down 30° below the horizontal and turns it to one side. The patient then sits up, is asked to report any sensation of dizziness and is observed for nystagmus. The manoeuvre is repeated for the right and left side in turn. The provocation of vertigo without nystagmus suggests benign positional vertigo. The provocation of vertigo with nystagmus on one or other side suggests cerebellar disease on that side. Provocation of vertigo on tilting below the horizontal alone suggests cervical spondylosis with nipping of the basilar artery, which can also occur on looking directly upwards.

Postural hypotension is suggested by symptoms occurring on arising or on getting up from recumbent or seated positions. It is confirmed by measurement of blood pressure in both seated and standing positions. Anxiety as a cause of dizziness is often considered after vertigo has been ruled out but may also be suggested by other symptoms and signs of anxiety – particularly hyperventilation (in which the associated hypocapnia may be the main factor inducing dizziness).

The presence of other ear symptoms, particularly tinnitus and/or deafness, suggests labyrinthine disease rather than cerebellar disease. Likewise, the presence of more general neurological disturbance, such as weaknesses or paraesthesias, suggests cerebellar disease.

Management

If there is evidence of cerebellar disease or labyrinthine disease further assessment and investigation are often required to identify the precise cause and so referral will be the usual response in a general practice setting. However, if there are indications of an acute self-limiting cause (such as labyrinthitis associated with a cold in a younger patient) or of benign disease such as benign positional vertigo, or of anxiety as the most probable cause, the condition may be managed symptomatically. Symptomatic treatments for vertigo include cyclizine and prochlorperazine. Use of neck collar may be helpful in cervical spondylosis. If postural hypotension is related to anti-hypertensive treatment this may need to be adjusted, otherwise improvement in symptoms can be achieved by modification to lifestyle and avoidance of sudden changes in position.

Collapse

The acute situation of finding a patient collapsed or unconscious is dealt with in Chapter 3. This section deals with the more common situation where a patient attends a GP saying they have had one or more episodes of collapse. See Box 4.32.

Diagnostic pointers

A vasovagal attack is usually presaged by a period of light-headedness and a feeling of things turning dark. Rapid recovery, especially once collapse has occurred, is the norm. The attack is sometimes provoked by some sort of psychogenic shock. In previously undiagnosed epilepsy a third-party history is very important and would confirm the

Box 4.32   Causes of collapse

Likely	**Possible**
Simple faint (vasovagal attack)	TIA/stroke
Epilepsy	Space occupying brain lesions (e.g. brain tumour)
Stokes–Adams attack(s) (elderly especially)/ Cardiac arrhythmia	Conversion reactions (hysteria)
Alcohol/ drug intoxication	Aortic stenosis
Anxiety (± hyperventilation)	Atypical migraine
	Addison's disease

occurrence of tonic–clonic movements and other features of epilepsy. Injury caused during the episode of collapse also makes epilepsy more likely.

'Stokes–Adams attack' is a name given to the phenomenon that occurs most typically in elderly patients where they suddenly drop to the ground without warning. Recovery is usually quite rapid. They are associated with a variety of cardiac problems, particularly arrhythmias, which will usually be detected on ECG. In younger patients, too, episodes of collapse can be associated with cardiac rhythm disturbances.

Alcohol and drugs are common causes of collapse and recurrent collapse and, surprisingly, patients do not ascribe their falling down to their drugs or alcohol. Anxiety will usually be obvious from other features and collapse is more likely to ensue in circumstances in which hyperventilation occurs. Stroke or transient ischaemic attack (TIA) may present with collapse but will usually be accompanied by more obvious signs such as unilateral paraplegia. Other causes may only become apparent over time or in hospital.

104

Management

In most instances of non-acute collapse presenting to GPs the task is to rule out serious causes for the complaint and, if this can be done, to reassure the patient. In the case of cardiac arrhythmias a precise diagnosis of the type of arrhythmia is very important as treatment varies according to this. Patients suffering a TIA will need some form of anti-platelet treatment such as aspirin to reduce the risk of further TIA or progression to stroke. For most of the other causes of collapse specialist advice will be required.

Numbness/altered sensation
See Box 4.33 for causes.

Diagnostic pointers

Numbness or paraesthesia confined to one part of the body suggests a local cause, e.g. trauma or compression, while

Box 4.33   Causes of numbness

Likely
Anxiety (esp. with
    hyperventilation)
Nerve compression
    syndromes
Carpal tunnel
Sciatica
Cervical spondylosis
Prolapsed or slipped discs

Possible
Diabetic neuropathy
Multiple sclerosis
Peripheral neuropathy (e.g.
    related to drugs, alcohol,
    B12 deficiency etc.)
Stroke/TIA
Syringomyelia
CNS tumours (spinal cord
    or brain)
Conversion reactions
    (hysteria)

more generalised paraesthesia is suggestive of more systemic disease or upset. Anxiety can be either but, if localised, the area of altered sensation may show a non-anatomical distribution i.e. not related to any specific nerves (e.g. stocking or glove distribution). Cervical spondylosis causes problems through compression of nerve roots. The same phenomenon gives rise to sciatica but the involved roots are typically lumbar or sacral. If there is acute nerve compression of spinal nerve roots, as occurs in slipped or prolapsed intervertebral discs, there is usually considerable pain as well.

Management

Altered sensation is an indicator of potentially serious problems and so a thorough investigation into the cause, involving specialists if necessary, is merited. Treatment is then specific to the cause.

Eye symptoms

Red eye
See Box 4.34 for causes.

Box 4.34   Causes of red-eye

Likely
Conjunctivitis

- infective
- allergic

Subconjunctival
  haemorrhage,
  haematoma

Possible
Acute glaucoma
Episcleritis/scleritis
Iritis (anterior uveitis)
Keratoconjunctivitis sicca
  (dry eye)
Keratitis/corneal ulcer
Intraocular foreign body

Diagnostic pointers

Acute onset associated with purulent discharge/sticky eye but with irritation, itchiness, or grittiness rather than pain and no impairment of visual acuity is suggestive of infective conjunctivitis. If it occurs in the context of an upper airways infection it is almost certainly viral but the more severe the eye symptoms and the more purulent the discharge the more likely it is to be bacterial. Less severe but more persistent symptoms may be suggestive of an allergic conjunctivitis – as is a failure to settle after a course of antibiotic eye drops or ointment. Again if symptoms are seasonal or associated with other features of hay fever an allergic cause is also more likely.

Subconjunctival haemorrhage has a characteristic appearance in which there is a localised very bright red (bloody) looking part of the eye affected. It may be induced by a sudden increase in intraocular pressure such as during a particularly violent sneeze or following blunt trauma. It is important to check the visual acuity, which should be unaffected in an uncomplicated subconjunctival haematoma.

- Acute glaucoma presents with acute onset of a very painful red eye, which may be accompanied by nausea or even vomiting. Vision is impaired and the affected eye has a fixed semi-dilated and cloudy pupil and the eye feels hard.
- Episcleritis and scleritis are localised inflammations of the eye beneath the conjunctiva. Episcleritis is more

localised and more likely to be self-limiting. They are not associated with discharge but there is usually a lot of reflex lacrimation.

- Acute iritis (or anterior uveitis) is suggested by redness around the cornea and a small, poorly reactive pupil and blurring of vision but without any discharge.
- Keratoconjunctivitis sicca or dry eye is a condition that is common in the elderly and in various connective tissue disorders such as Sjogren's syndrome. It is associated with a dry gritty feeling in the eyes but no discharge and no effect on vision.
- Keratitis or corneal ulcer is suggested by very painful red eye associated with blurred vision. The patient will not usually be able to open the eye and may complain of extreme photophobia. The damage to the cornea will be revealed by vital dye (e.g. fluorescein) staining – the damaged area showing up as green stained with fluorescein. Symptoms overlap with those of a penetrating foreign body and both may be associated with trauma.

Management

Bacterial conjunctivitis is usually treated with anti-bacterial eye drops such as chloramphenicol 0.5% or fusidic acid 1%. Viral conjunctivitis strictly speaking does not need specific treatment although, in practice, because of the practical difficulty in distinguishing it from bacterial conjunctivitis it is often treated with anti-bacterial drops. Allergic conjunctivitis is managed by reducing exposure to the allergen if it can be identified and avoided; otherwise treatment is with sodium cromoglycate eye drops, although anti-histamines can also be helpful and may manage other co-existing allergic symptoms e.g. in hay fever. Subconjunctival haemorrhage does not require any local treatment and the patient usually just needs to be reassured about the benign nature of this condition. If persistent or recurrent it is advisable to investigate the patient for a bleeding diathesis.

- Acute glaucoma is a sight-threatening emergency and needs urgent (usually in-patient) treatment with intravenous acetazolamide and pilocarpine eye drops to constrict the pupil.
- Scleritis and episcleritis are usually treated with corticosteroid eye drops but care must be taken to rule out a herpes keratitis as steroids applied to an eye with a 'dendritic ulcer' can lead to profound damage to the cornea and blindness.
- Iritis is often related to other conditions such as various autoimmune diseases and the underlying cause of the condition needs to be found and treated. The eye condition may also need treatment with corticosteroid drops and dilation of the pupil e.g. with atropine.
- Simple dry eye conditions are treated with 'artificial tears' such as hypromellose eye drops.
- Keratitis or corneal abrasions are treated with anti-bacterial eye drops (primarily to prevent bacterial super-infection) and the eye is padded for 24–48 hours. However, if the keratitis is associated with herpes zoster (as in zoster ophthalmitis) the pattern of damage on fluorescein staining is that of a 'dendritic ulcer' and it will require anti-viral treatment (e.g. with aciclovir drops) and papillary dilatation with atropine. This should be undertaken under specialist supervision.

Defects of vision (blurring or loss of vision)

See Box 4.35 for causes.

Diagnostic pointers

As is obvious from the categories above, whether the onset is sudden or gradual it is crucial to distinguishing the cause of visual defects. The patient's age is another important factor with certain conditions such as cataract, senile macular degeneration, temporal arteritis and chronic glaucoma becoming progressively more likely with advancing years and highly improbable in the young. Several conditions affecting vision are not primarily eye diseases (such as diabetes, stroke and migraine) and extraocular features will probably lead one to the cause in these conditions.

Box 4.35 Causes of blurring or loss of vision

Likely
Gradual onset

- refractive errors (long or short sightedness)
- cataract
- chronic glaucoma
- diabetes
- hypertensive retinopathy
- senile macular degeneration

Acute onset

- acute glaucoma
- vitreous haemorrhage
- central retinal arterial occlusion
- migraine
- TIA/stroke

Possible
Gradual onset

- optic neuritis e.g. in multiple sclerosis
- choroidoretinitis
- retinitis pigmentosa
- intraorbital or intracranial tumours
- toxic amblyopia (e.g. due to drugs such as tobacco, methanol, or quinine)

Acute onset

- central retinal vein occlusion
- retrobulbar neuritis
- retinal detachment
- temporal arteritis
- posterior uveitis
- cortical blindness
- hysterical blindness

109

Otherwise the appearance of the eye and/or fundus will reveal the cause – further details will be found in textbooks of ophthalmology or of clinical examination.

Management

There are a large number of conditions associated with visual impairment and the management of these will be specific to the cause. Consult general ophthalmology or medicine texts for details.

Skin symptoms

Virtually all skin diseases present with a rash. Rashes can be categorised according to the appearance of principle lesion comprising the rash. The main lesions found in rashes are:

- erythema
- macules
- papules
- pustules
- vesicles and/or bullae
- scales and plaques
- itch (pruritis)
- nodules
- purpura and/or petechiae.

Vesicles and bullae are produced by the same sorts of disease process, bullae really just being enlarged vesicles and so these are considered together. Similarly, purpura are really just large petechiae. Conditions that produce scales can also produce plaques (i.e. raised areas of skin) and conditions associated with either are considered together.

Erythematous rashes

See Box 4.36 for causes of these types of rash.

Diagnostic pointers

Cellulitis is due to an infection of the deep subcutaneous layer and so the affected area (often in the lower limb) will

---

Box 4.36   Causes of erythematous rashes

Likely	**Possible**
Cellulitis	Erythema multiforme
Erysipelas	Erythema ab igne
Gout	Erythema nodosum
Drug reaction	Systemic lupus
Bacterial infections (e.g.	erythematosus
scarlet fever)	Photosensitivity (e.g.
Viral infection (measles)	phenothiazines)
Sun burn	

be hot to the touch and the patient may be pyrexial and unwell too. Erysipelas is the name given to a more superficial form of cellulitis. Lesions are shiny red and well demarcated. Gout typically affects joints, especially the metatarso-phalangeal joint of the hallux, and is associated with acute severe pain with redness and increased temperature at the joint.

Drug reactions produce a great variety of rashes including generalised erythema, more localised erythema at specific sites and erythema nodosum and erythema multiforme (see below). A great many viral and several bacterial infections (particularly streptococcal infections) may be associated with various intensities of erythema. Many rashes such as the morbilliform rash of measles, the bright red cheeks of fifth disease and the widespread erythema but circumoral pallor of scarlet fever are characteristic of the particular infections but others are non-specific and are recognised by their association with other more general features of the associated systemic infection.

The association with exposure to bright sunlight is usually recognised in cases of sunburn, although sometimes the patient will have overlooked it as a cause of a bright red rash. The distribution in areas of skin exposed to the sun will also raise the suspicion. Erythema nodosum appears as tender dark bluish red nodules on the shins or lower limbs. Erythema multiforme also has a characteristic polycyclic, annular or 'target lesion' appearance. Both of these conditions are associated with a number of other underlying conditions – for further details consult a textbook of dermatology. Erythema ab igne is a dark red or brawny rash with a reticulate appearance caused by prolonged exposure of skin to an open fire. It typically occurs in lower limbs in older patients who keep warm by sitting in front of a fire.

Systemic lupus erythematosus is associated with a characteristic facial rash described as having a 'butterfly' distribution on the cheeks. Photosensitive rashes, which may occur in patients on photosensitising drugs such as phenothiazines, are associated with widespread erythema following even quite brief exposure to sunlight. Distribution in areas exposed to sunlight is an important indicator.

Management

Cellulitis and erysipelas are treated with appropriate antibiotics – usually penicillin V or flucloxacillin. Acute gout is
treated with a potent non-steroidal anti-inflammatory such
as indomethacin, providing the patient is suitable for this
kind of drug. Most viral infections do not require any specific treatment but bacterial infections such as scarlet fever
need treatment with appropriate antibiotics. Other rashes
are treated depending on their cause and readers are
referred to textbooks of medicine or dermatology for further
details.

Macular rashes
See Box 4.37.

Diagnostic pointers

Macules are flat, circumscribed areas of discoloration of the
skin. Widespread small red macules occur in the presence
of many viral infections, especially in small children, and
are a non-specific indicator of viral illnesses. A similar
widespread distribution of small red macules can be a drug
reaction – the accompanying history of drug consumption
being the key to distinguishing these conditions. In chloasma
lesions are larger and brownish in colour and occur typically on the face. It is associated with pregnancy but may
sometimes be induced by the oral contraceptive pill. Moles
may be raised (i.e. papular) but are often macules of various
sizes in various locations in varying shades of brown. Moles

112

Box 4.37 Causes of macular rashes

Likely	Possible
Non-specific viral exanthema	Measles
	Rubella
Drug reaction	Café-au-lait spots
Chloasma	Pityriasis versicolor
Moles (naevus)	Pityriasis alba

that have well demarcated boundaries and are not undergoing change are usually benign.

In other conditions associated with macules, such as measles and rubella, the macular rash is only part of a usually well-recognised syndrome, the other features of which enable the condition to be identified. 'Café-au-lait spots' are, as the name suggests, light brown patches. They may occur anywhere on the body and are associated with neurofibromatosis. Pityriasis versicolor is a fungal infection associated with variably pigmented lesions on different areas of the body – exposed areas of the body may have lesions that are lighter than surrounding skin whereas areas not exposed to sunlight may have lesions that are slightly darker than surrounding skin. Pityriasis alba is a form of eczema associated with paler-coloured macules, especially on the face, in children.

Management

Viral illnesses, either non-specific or specific ones such as measles, are treated largely symptomatically with fluids and anti-pyretic measures primarily. Removing the offending drug is, obviously, the way to counter drug reactions, although a re-challenge may sometimes be indicated to be sure of the diagnosis. However, such a re-challenge is potentially dangerous and would not normally be undertaken in general practice. Pityriasis versicolor is treated with antifungals and pityriasis alba is treated as per other forms of eczema (see below).

Papular rashes
See Box 4.38 for the causes.

Diagnostic pointers

Papules are small raised lesions. They are often associated with a surrounding redness in maculopapular rashes. If they contain pus they are called pustules (see next section). Larger elevated lesions (larger than 5 cm) are called nodules

Box 4.38 Causes of papular rashes

Likely	**Possible**
Acne	Insect bites
Scabies	Milia (babies)
Viral wart	Seborrhoeic wart
Non-specific viral rash	Guttate psoriasis
	Lichen planus
	Prickly heat
	Malignant melanoma
	Kaposi's sarcoma
	Acanthosis nigricans

(see below) although if they become vesicular they may develop into blisters or bullae (see below).

Acne vulgaris is recognisable from its distribution on face and upper arms and trunk and its association with adolescence, although it may persist into adulthood – especially in women. The lesions of scabies also have a typical distribution, affecting areas of the body from the neck down, but are even more strongly characterised by their intense itch, especially at night.

Warts have a characteristic cruciferous (cauliflower-like) appearance although they may be flatter and smoother in areas of the body where they are under pressure (such as on the feet, where they are called 'verrucae'). They vary in size and may appear in clumps. As noted above, viral infections can cause a great variety of rashes including maculopapular or even just papular lesions. Insect bites, like scabies, are itchy but are more localised. Seborrhoeic warts are associated with other features of seborrhoea, especially scaling.

In guttate psoriasis the papules are red and may be dispersed throughout the body. They may also become vesicular. Lichen planus is associated with flat-topped papules with a shiny surface and occasionally white streaks called Wickham's striae. Common sites are the wrists, arms and legs. Prickly heat is also red and itchy and is characterised by its association with excessive heat.

Malignant melanoma typically develops from pigmented moles that undergo change – becoming larger, darker or more varied in colour, or beginning to itch or bleed or developing an irregular or poorly defined margin. Kaposi's sarcoma is associated with the later stages of AIDS. Lesions are polychromatic and vary in size and are typically found on the face, palate, trunk, limbs and oral mucosa. They may develop into plaques. In acanthosis nigricans there are hyperpigmented papules most commonly in the axillae, limb flexures and backs of the hands and neck. It is associated with various internal malignancies.

Management

Acne is managed initially with topical treatments, especially benzoyl peroxide. There are a variety of other topical treatments used including sulphur and salicylate containing treatments, and vitamin A based treatments. If, after an adequate trial, topical treatments do not clear the acne, long-term antibiotics may be used either topically or orally. Tetracyclines are effective but contraindicated in women of child-bearing age unless the patient is on reliable contraception. For women, or men who do not respond to tetracyclines, erythromycin topically or orally and clindamycin topically are alternatives. In women the anti-oestrogen cyproterone acetate is another option – it is given in combination with ethinyloestradiol, which acts as a contraceptive, in co-cyprindiol. Retinoids are used in severe cases but this is a specialist treatment.

Scabies may be treated with a lotion of either malathion or permethrin, which is applied from the neck down and left on overnight before washing off. All intimate contacts should be treated simultaneously.

Warts are usually treated initially with a salicylate or lactic acid preparation applied to the wart daily with abrasion of the wart between treatments, e.g. with a pumice stone or emery board. Liquid nitrogen is another form of treatment commonly used where facilities for such cryotherapy are available. Podophyllin is a treatment used for the treatment of genital warts. There are various other treatments but for all treatments many applications may be necessary as relapse after treatment is common.

Pustular rashes

See Box 4.39 for causes.

Diagnostic pointers

The development of pus is a product of inflammation but is typically associated with infection. In the skin pustules are, likewise, indicative of active inflammation involving leukocytes and are mostly a manifestation of infection. In non-bullous impetigo there are pustules with typical crusts. In folliculitis there are small non-crusting pustules with surrounding erythema. Sycosis barbae is a form of folliculitis occurring in the beard area. The typical distribution of lesions of acne on the face, neck and upper trunk has been mentioned above. Pustules are a more advanced manifestation of the condition.

The lesions of rosacea also have a typical distribution on the cheeks and forehead but occur more often in older adults. It may be associated with rhinophyma. Herpes simplex and zoster usually start with vesicles and progress to pustules which later crust. Hidradenitis suppurativa is a condition associated with excessive sweat production in which areas of the body with lots of sweat glands, such as the axillae, may become infected, producing pustules and furuncles that are very persistent.

Box 4.39   Causes of pustular rashes

Likely	**Possible**
Impetigo	Hidradenitis suppurativa
Folliculitis	Dermatitis herpetiformis
Sycosis barbae	Behcet's syndrome
Acne vulgaris	Drug-induced
Rosacea	
Herpes simplex	
Herpes zoster	

Dermatitis herpetiformis more typically presents with vesicles but these may progress to pustules. It may show a typical distribution pattern of the extensor surfaces of elbows and knees and the back and buttocks. It occurs in early and middle adult life and may be associated with coeliac disease. Behcet's syndrome is an autoimmune condition in which a wide variety of skin lesions may occur, including pustules. Oral ulceration and eye complications are common manifestations of this difficult to recognise and manage condition. As noted above, drug reactions are capable of inducing most manifestations of skin disease, including pustules, which may be distinguishable from their widespread rather than localised presentation.

Management

Impetigo and folliculitis are treated with antibiotics active against the commonest organism associated with this condition, namely *Staphylococcus aureus*. In milder and less extensive cases topical preparations may suffice but in more extensive disease, or if topical preparations fail, oral antibiotics may be required. The management of acne is covered above. Rosacea is also treated with long-term oral tetracyclines. Some of the topical treatments used in acne such as benzoyl peroxide may also be useful. Hidradenitis suppurativa is usually treated initially with antibiotics such as flucloxacillin but in severe or persistent cases surgery may be required. Dermatitis herpetiformis is treated with dapsone or sulphapyridine in addition to a gluten-free diet. Colchicine is used as an initial treatment for Behcet's syndrome. Steroids and immunosuppressants are also used in management. Further details are beyond the scope of this book.

Vesicular (and/or bullous) rashes

See Box 4.40 for causes of these types of rash.

Diagnostic pointers

Diseases that produce vesicles (or blisters) overlap substantially with those that produce bullae, which are simple

Box 4.40   Causes of vesicular/bullous rashes

Likely	Possible
Herpes simplex	Pemphigus
Herpes zoster (chickenpox or shingles)	Pemphigoid
	Dermatitis herpetiformis
Hand-foot-mouth disease (children)	Bullous impetigo
	Drug reaction
Eczema (esp. pompholyx)	Erythema multiforme
	Porphyria
	Toxic epidermal necrolysis
	Epidermolysis bullae

vesicles larger than 0.5 cm. Blistering conditions can be distinguished by the three D's – development, duration and distribution. The development of vesicles in the presence of more generalised illness is typically associated with viral illnesses such as chickenpox and hand-foot-mouth disease. Vesicles developing quickly are associated with allergies and infections such as in drug reactions and impetigo. Localised blistering is associated with eczema, allergic reactions, insect bites, psoriasis, impetigo and herpes simplex and shingles (which is a manifestation of a recrudescence of herpes zoster). Other conditions associated with vesicle formation tend to be more widespread.

Herpes simplex type I occurs initially in childhood and is most commonly seen on the face, lips and buccal mucosa. It may later recrudesce as 'cold sores'. Herpes simplex type II is a sexually transmitted infection that presents with intensely itchy and painful lesions in the genital area. Primary infection with herpes zoster (chickenpox) presents with crops of itchy lesions in different areas of the body, which are initially erythematous, then develop vesicles, then pustules and then crusts. Oral lesions may also occur. In secondary infection (shingles) crops of vesicles appear in a dermatome distribution on either the trunk or a branch of the trigeminal nerve. The appearance of the shingles rash may be preceded by pain or paraesthesia in the affected area. In hand-foot-mouth disease vesicles occur in the areas suggested by the name, prodromal viral symptoms also occur. Eczema is more typically a dry scaly rash (see below) but certain manifestations – especially pompholyx – are associated with vesicles. In pompholyx typical sites for vesicles are palms of the hands, soles of the feet and fingers.

Pemphigus and pemphigoid are two easily confused conditions as both are associated with widespread bullae occurring in adults. Distinguishing features include the fact that bullae in pemphigus are more friable, the mucous membranes may be affected, the presence of Nikolsky's sign (i.e. even just rubbing the skin causes the epidermis to slough off), and younger patients tend to be affected. Pemphigoid is a disease of elderly people, which can relapse and remit. Lesions (which are less friable than in pemphigus) occur in more confined distribution on arms and legs. Pemphigus is a life threatening illness. Dermatitis herpetiformis has been mentioned above as it may progress to pustules; also, it tends to be more vesicular than bullous. Bullous impetigo is a form of impetigo associated with widespread bullae, which may become pus filled and may rupture, leaving crusts. Typical sites are face and limbs and typical sufferers are young children.

The typical lesion of erythema multiforme is the 'target lesion' (described above) but vesicles or bullae may also develop. Stevens–Johnson syndrome is a manifestation of erythema multiforme associated with severe bullous lesions and lesions of the mucous membranes. Porphyria is a genetic disorder – one of the manifestations is blistering of the skin on minimal exposure to sunlight or from minor trauma. Toxic epidermal necrolysis is associated with the rapid onset of widespread bullous disease similar to but much more rapid in onset than pemphigus. As in pemphigus, skin easily sloughs off (Nikolsky's sign). It is often associated with drug ingestion and is considered by some as a very severe form of erythema multiforme or Stevens–Johnson syndrome (see above). It can be rapidly fatal. Epidermolysis bullae is a rare congenital condition that can occur in varying degrees of severity. It is associated with spontaneous blister or bulla formation occurring from birth. In milder forms bullae do not so readily occur and healing occurs without scarring. In more severe forms scarring does occur and contractural deformities may result.

Management

Herpes simplex infections may be treated with aciclovir cream. Chickenpox does not usually require specific remedies but is treated with symptomatic remedies such as calamine lotion. More severe or recurrent herpetic infections are treated with oral antivirals but these must be given early in the development of symptoms to be of much benefit. Treatment of eczema is dealt with below (see dry scaly rashes). The mainstay of treatment of both pemphigus and pemphigoid is oral steroids but immunosuppressants such as azathioprine are also often used (especially in pemphigus). Treatment of dermatitis herpetiformis comprises dapsone and gluten-free diet. Bullous impetigo, as with other forms, is treated with antibiotics but oral treatment is more likely to be required. The key to the management of erythema multiforme is the removal of any cause that can be identified, such as a drug. In more severe manifestations, such as Stevens–Johnson syndrome and toxic epidermal necrolysis, oral corticosteroids may be used.

Dry scaly rashes
See Box 4.41 for causes of these types of rash.

Diagnostic pointers

Eczema is an inflammatory condition of skin that can show many different manifestations. Dry scaling itchy skin affecting particularly flexor surfaces is the typical presentation of atopic eczema. Contact dermatitis is another manifestation in which dry scaly itchy skin occurs in areas in contact with an allergen. Dry scaly skin occurring in areas of the body with many sebaceous glands such as the scalp, face, and eyebrows is called seborrhoeic dermatitis – it is another manifestation of eczema. Lichen simplex is yet another manifestation of eczema in which lichenification (thicken-

Box 4.41   Causes of a dry/scaly rash

Likely	**Possible**
Psoriasis	Lichen simplex
Eczema	Lichen planus
Tinea infections	Solar keratosis
Seborrhoeic dermatitis	Pityriasis versicolor
	Pityriasis rosea
	Bowen's disease
	Mycosis fungoides
	Drug-induced (beta blockers, carbamazepine)

ing of the skin with increased markings) predominates in localised patches.

Psoriasis is associated with well-demarcated raised plaques of erythematous skin covered in thick silvery-white scales. Scales, which may be removable, tend to thicken over time – underlying skin is typically shiny, red, and smooth. Typical distribution is on the extensor surfaces (elbows and knees) and on the scalp, sacral area, chest, face, abdomen and genitalia. Psoriasis is a hereditary condition and so there is often a family history. Psoriasis also shows the Koebner phenomenon, in which lesions develop at the site of injuries. Nails may also be involved with pitting, splitting and thickening. There may be an associated arthropathy.

Ringworm is a common type of fungal skin infection in which lesions are well demarcated with a slowly extending scaly margin with apparent clearing at the centre. They may occur in many different sites. Erythema with scaling in the groin areas, tinea cruris, is another manifestation of fungal infection.

Lesions of lichen planus are well defined, raised and may have a scaly surface and resemble psoriasis. They may also display the Koebner phenomenon (see above). However, the lesions of lichen planus are usually itchy, they may have the characteristic Wickham's striae and they occur on flexor aspects of limbs.

121

Solar or actinic keratoses are raised, sometimes hyper-pigmented, lesions with a crumbling surface typically seen in older patients on areas of skin exposed to sunlight. They may become dysplastic and progress to squamous cell carcinomas.

Pityriasis versicolor is described above as a variably pigmented macular rash but it may also appear dry and scaly – which is indicative of its fungal aetiology. Pityriasis rosea presents initially with a single annular patch that is reddish brown with a raised edge. The first patch to appear is called the 'herald patch' and others soon follow – typically on the trunk, neck and upper parts of limbs. Pityriasis rosea may be accompanied by mild sore throat and generalised malaise. Bowen's disease presents with a single well-defined erythematous or reddish brown macule with crusting or scaling. It is histologically a carcinoma-in-situ.

The lesions of mycosis fungoides are initially well-demarcated erythematous scaly patches (quite similar to psoriasis) that are intensely itchy (which lesions of psoriasis are typically not) and occur in non-exposed areas of the body. Mycosis fungoides is actually a type of T-cell lymphoma occurring in the skin. Drugs can also produce scaly rashes, which may resemble eczema (i.e. with erythema, scaling and poorly defined lesions) or psoriasis (with well defined plaques).

Management

Dry scaly forms of eczema should be treated with emollients and steroid ointments. Wet or weeping lesions should be treated with wet soaks and wraps and steroid creams. Topical steroids need to be used with care because of the danger of an irreversible thinning of the skin that can occur if they are overused. Eczema is commonly complicated by secondary infection and topical or, in severe cases, oral antibiotics may also be needed. Contact dermatitis will also be helped if the offending allergen can be identified and contact avoided. Patch testing may be useful in this regard. A topical preparation of an immunosuppressant drug, tacrolimus, has recently become available for the treatment of eczema. Its place in therapy has not yet been fully identified.

Coal tar preparations and salicylic acid may be useful in mild, limited and stable psoriasis. Ichthammol is another alternative. Dithranol is another topical preparation that is more effective for thicker lichenified lesions but it must be applied with care as it is very irritant to healthy skin. Topical corticosteroids are also effective at clearing psoriasis but there is often relapse when they are withdrawn and tachyphylaxis may develop. Oral steroids are only used in erythroderma as rebound is almost inevitable. Calcipotriol and tacalcitol are vitamin D analogues that are also useful in plaque psoriasis. Ultraviolet B (UVB) treatment is useful for widespread thin lesions or guttate psoriasis but ultraviolet A in combination with psoralen (PUVA) is an alternative phototherapy used to clear or reduce psoriasis in severe cases. Extensive or severe psoriasis may also be treated with systemic anti-metabolite or immunosuppressant treatments including methotrexate, azathioprine, hydroxyurea and ciclosporin. Acitretin is another hospital-only systemic therapy – it is a vitamin A derivative.

Fungal skin infections are treated initially with topical antifungal creams such as clotrimazole. In more resistant cases systemic antifungals may be used – but this should only be on the basis of mycobiological testing.

Mild lichen planus may not need any treatment but the associated itching is often relieved by moderately potent steroid ointments. In severe or widespread disease a course of oral steroids may be prescribed.

Solar keratoses may be treated with liquid nitrogen or curettage. Pityriasis versicolor is treated with selenium sulphide. Pityriasis rosea does not require any specific treatment but calamine lotion or mild topical steroids may relieve any accompanying itch. Bowen's disease may be treated with cryotherapy. Mycosis fungoides requires specialist treatment.

Purpuric rashes

See Box 4.42.

123

Box 4.42 Causes of purpuric rash

Likely	**Possible**
Trauma (bruising)	Liver disease
Senile purpura	Drugs (e.g. warfarin, aspirin, steroids)
	Henoch–Schönlein purpura (children)
	Thrombocytopenia
	Renal failure
	Infective endocarditis
	Meningococcal septicaemia
	Bleeding diathesis e.g. Christmas disease, haemophilia

Diagnostic pointers

The most worrisome purpuric rash is that which occurs with meningococcal septicaemia. It progresses usually quite rapidly from a red to purplish coloured rash covering ever-larger areas of the body and occurs in an obviously ill patient who may also be showing signs of meningitis. Its non-blanching character may be useful in distinguishing it from other macular rashes. The basis of purpura is extravasation of blood under the skin. Hence it may occur after trauma (in bruises) and in older patients with thin skin and fragile subcutaneous blood vessels (senile purpura). It is also a feature of various bleeding disorders including bleeding diatheses secondary to liver, renal or bone marrow diseases. It may also occur in patients on anti-coagulants, anti-platelet drugs and corticosteroids. In Henoch–Schönlein purpura there is a purpuric eruption on the legs and buttocks and an associated nephritis. In infective endocarditis the purpura takes the form of small splinter haemorrhages in the nailbeds.

Management

Purpura is symptomatic of various systemic conditions rather than being a strictly dermatological condition. Details of the management of the myriad potential causes of purpura are beyond the scope of this book.

Itch (pruritis)

Causes are outlined in Box 4.43

Diagnostic pointers

Itch is a characteristic of many skin diseases that are more often distinguished on the basis of the lesions and their development, duration and distribution. It is an almost invariable feature of eczema but only occasionally a feature of psoriasis. Intense itching, especially at night, should always lead to a consideration of possible scabies.

Intense itching is also characteristic of urticaria but the typical weal and flare of urticaria lesions are more diagnostic. It should be remembered that itch, especially in the absence of an obvious rash, can be indicative of systemic illnesses such as liver disease (with or without jaundice), renal disease, and leukaemia or lymphoma. Itch with or without accompanying rash can also occur in drug reactions.

Management

Treatment of any underlying cause is obviously important in the management of itching (pruritus). Topical treatment

---

Box 4.43   *Causes of pruritus*

Likely	**Possible**
Eczema	Psoriasis
Contact dermatitis	Liver disease (esp. with jaundice)
Scabies	
Pityriasis rosea	Renal failure
Urticaria	Lichen planus
Chickenpox (in children)	Prickly heat
	Leukaemia
	Hodgkin's lymphoma
	Drug reaction

with calamine lotion, camphor-containing preparations, or crotamiton (Eurax) may be effective. Topical steroids, possibly with occlusive dressings, may also help. Antihistamines are also helpful and widely used.

Lumps on or just beneath the skin (nodules)

Likely and possible causes of nodules are listed in Box 4.44.

Diagnostic pointers

Lumps appearing anywhere on the body are often a source of alarm for patients who associate lumps automatically with malignant disease – many malignant diseases may present with lumps as either a primary or secondary lesion. However there are also many common benign causes of cutaneous or subcutaneous lumps. These are often distinguished by their well-defined edges, lack of involvement of surrounding tissues, their colour and distribution.

Sebaceous cysts, for instance, are firm smooth lumps of variable sizes occurring typically in the hairy areas of the body such as the head, face, neck and back. Lipomata are generally largish (>5 cm) rather soft smooth lumps found all over the body but mostly on the trunk. Normal viral warts

Box 4.44 Causes of nodules

Likely	Possible
Sebaceous cyst	Basal cell carcinoma
Lipoma	Squamous cell carcinoma
Wart	Nodulocystic acne
Xanthoma	Gouty tophi
Lymphadenopathy	Rheumatoid nodules
	Kerato-acanthoma
	Pyogenic granuloma
	Malignant melanoma
	Polyarteritis nodosa
	Lymphoma
	Sarcoidosis

are recognisable from their raised rough surfaces. They are more common in children and typical sites include the hands and feet. On the soles of the feet they may be flattened and painful and are called verrucae. Warts also occur in the genital area – where they are usually acquired by sexual contact.

Xanthomata are often yellowish in colour and are associated with severe hyperlipidaemia. Typical sites include eyelids and extensor surfaces of limbs. Lymphadenopathy (i.e. enlargement of lymph glands) occurs in the sites of lymph nodes such as the neck, axillae and groin in response to a local focus of inflammation or infection. It may be generalised in certain systemic conditions such as infective mononucleosis (glandular fever) or lymphoma. Lymphadenopathy should resolve after the source of inflammation is resolved but persistent lymphadenopathy raises the suspicion of a more chronic condition such as tuberculosis or sarcoid, or a malignant condition such as lymphoma or secondary spread of another primary tumour.

All forms of skin cancer may present as lumps. Basal cell carcinomas present as firm nodules that later break down to form the typical 'rodent ulcer' with the typical rolled edge. Squamous cell carcinomas have a more variable appearance and often begin in pre-existing lesions of solar keratosis or Bowen's disease. The edges of squamous cell carcinomas are typically irregular and poorly defined. Malignant melanomata arise from pigmented naevi that undergo some form of notable change such as bleeding, changing colour, developing pain or itch.

Severe acne can progress to formation of cysts or nodules but the diagnosis will be apparent from the preceding history of acne.

Nodules appearing in the skin of patients with joint disease may be either gouty tophi or rheumatoid nodules. Gouty tophi appear on the ears, hand or extensor surfaces of limb joints. Rheumatoid nodules tend to occur over pressure points.

Kerato-acanthomata start as small papules that grow rapidly over a period of a few months to form a raised lesion with a keratotic centre. The face is a common site. Pyogenic granulomata also occur as single, rapidly developing, bright red, softish nodules, which often develop at the site of some previous trauma. They tend to bleed easily. The skin nodes of polyarteritis nodosa are a manifestation of the underlying vasculitis and so they tend to occur along the line of affected arteries. They may be purpuric or red.

Management

Where the diagnosis is not clear from other features of the disease or the appearance of the nodule itself, the safest course with many skin lumps is often excision biopsy. Where skin lumps are manifestations of systemic disease the underlying systemic disease should, obviously, be treated appropriately. The treatment of viral warts is dealt with above (see papular lesions).

Breast symptoms

Breast pain (mastalgia)

Causes of mastalgia are given in Box 4.45.

Diagnostic pointers

Breast pain occurring mainly in the premenstrual part of a woman's menstrual cycle is cyclical mastalgia. It may be

Box 4.45   Causes of mastalgia

Likely	Possible
Pregnancy	Breast cancer
Cyclical mastalgia	Fibroadenosis
Mastitis (in lactating women)	Puberty (in both males and females)
Breast abscess	Costochondritis
Cracked/inflamed nipple (in lactating women)	Shingles
	Angina

associated with other features of premenstrual syndrome. A more persistent breast pain may be due to fibroadenosis of the breast but in a woman of child-bearing years and amenorrhoea it may be a symptom of pregnancy. Lactating mothers also get breast pain, which, if localised to the areola and associated with the baby's latching onto the breast, may be due to cracked or inflamed nipples. If there is tender, red area on one or other breast this may be mastitis or possibly a breast abscess. During puberty both males and females may develop mastalgia. Breast cancer does not usually present with pain but most typically with a lump. However, in a woman presenting with breast pain and a lump cancer should be considered as a possible cause until it can be ruled out.

If the pain is not located in the breast itself it may be due to a musculoskeletal disease such as costochondritis. In older patients more sinister cardiovascular or respiratory disease may need to be considered, e.g. angina. In shingles the pain along a dermatome distribution may precede the onset of the rash and is a possible cause of diagnostic confusion.

Management

Cyclical mastalgia may be helped by non-steroidal anti-inflammatories or by gamalenic acid. Fibroadenosis of the breast may be helped by simple analgesics or NSAIDs but a well-fitting bra may also help relieve the problem. Cracked or inflamed nipples are treated with an emollient such as chamomile extract (Kamillosan) and by good breast-feeding technique, which may require the guidance of an experienced midwife or breast-feeding support worker. Mastitis and breast abscess are treated with antibiotics, although if an abscess fails to recede with antibiotic therapy surgical incision and drainage may be required. Treatment of conditions not specific to the breast is considered elsewhere.

Breast lump

Box 4.46 lists the causes of breast lumps.

Box 4.46 Causes of breast lumps

Likely	**Possible**
Fibroadenoma	Lipoma
Breast cyst	Paget's disease of the breast
Breast abscess	Fat necrosis
Carcinoma of the breast	Lymphoma

Diagnostic pointers

Fibroadenomata present typically in young women. They are well defined and usually highly mobile within the breast tissue. Breast cysts are also usually well defined and usually occur in women with diffusely 'lumpy' breasts characteristic of fibroadenosis. They are often diagnosed by the way they can be resolved by fine-needle aspiration. Breast abscesses are most common during lactation and are associated with preceding mastitis and the presence of a red, hot, very tender lump. Lipomata (see above under skin nodules) can present in the breast and may be recognisable by their rather soft feel. Fat necrosis of an area of the breast may occur after trauma and is recognised by bruising and discoloration of overlying skin.

The big worry in a woman presenting with a breast lump, though, is that it might be breast cancer. Any woman presenting with a breast lump for which a benign cause cannot easily be identified should be referred to a specialist breast cancer centre for assessment. The co-existence of a nipple discharge with a breast lump may represent Paget's disease of the breast, which is also a malignant condition and requires specialist management.

Management

Fibroadenomata, if they can be confidently diagnosed, need not be excised – but they often are. However, they recur and recurrent lesions need not be excised in young women.

Cysts are treated by aspiration but the aspirate must be checked for malignant cells. Treatment of breast abscesses is dealt with above. Fat necrosis resolves spontaneously and usually does not need active treatment. The treatment of breast cancer is a highly specialised area so patients suspected of this condition must be referred.

Nipple discharge

See Box 4.47.

Diagnostic pointers

Amenorrhoea in a woman of child-bearing years is the telltale feature of pregnancy, even if the initial presentation is one of nipple discharge. Breast abscesses are hot and painful and occur typically in lactating mothers. In duct ectasia part of the breast may also become tender and indurated and there is a thick, toothpaste-like discharge. Paget's disease of the nipple gives rise to a discharge, which may be bloody. There is crusting and scaling of the nipple but there is not always a lump so nipple discharge in an older woman requires a biopsy for diagnosis. Intraductal carcinoma may present with a discharge but there will usually be a lump present too, although it may require mammography to identify it. Hyperprolactinoma can be due to drugs as well as pituitary tumours. Galactorrhoea is a characteristic feature. Other features are amenorrhoea, subfertility, low libido and headaches and/or visual field defects where it is due to a pituitary tumour.

Box 4.47   Causes of nipple discharge

Likely	**Possible**
Pregnancy	Paget's disease of the breast
Duct ectasia	Intraductal carcinoma
Breast abscess	Hyperprolactinoma

Management

Virtually all causes of a nipple discharge, except normal lactation, pregnancy and puberty, have potentially sinister implications and will usually require referral to a specialist.

Psychological symptoms

Anxiety

Virtually any symptom known can be attributed to anxiety and virtually any symptom can induce a degree of anxiety in patients. However, patients presenting with a feeling of anxiety as their main complaint are relatively few. Symptoms are often attributed to anxiety when they cannot be attributed to a recognisable physical disorder. However, this is potentially dangerously misleading and it is important in making the diagnosis of anxiety as an explanation for physical symptoms that you also try to identify positive features of anxiety. Note also that, in addition to generalised anxiety disorder (sometimes called 'free floating' anxiety), there are a number of more specific anxiety disorders including phobic anxiety (which include a larger number of specific phobias), panic disorder, and obsessive–compulsive disorder.

Diagnostic pointers

Anxiety is associated with outpouring of adrenalin (the classic 'fight or flight' response) and so is associated with symptoms of sympathetic activity including breathlessness, palpitations, increased sweating, feelings of emptiness or fluttering in the stomach, tremulousness and so on. At higher levels of intensity it may be associated with other symptoms such as nausea, vomiting, diarrhoea, muscle aches and insomnia. Patients with anxiety or stress will often admit to feeling anxious if asked, although they may be reluctant to confess to anxiety if they feel this will lead

132

to them being taken less seriously or to their symptoms being dismissed as not 'real'.

Sometimes, even though the patient denies feelings of anxiety or stress, it is still apparent from their demeanour – they may look pale, they may be wringing their hands or handling other objects in a restless manner, they may be restless or wary looking, and they may talk very fast and range widely over topics. Patients with anxiety will often have a pre-morbid tendency to worry easily and excessively, and perhaps a history of anxiety or anxiety-related disorders (such as phobias, obsessive–compulsive disorder etc.).

Possible causes

Anxiety is a natural response to situations that are threatening or perceived as threatening. Where there is actual threat it is, of course, an adaptive response, but more often the threat is more perceived than real. The sources of perceived threat are myriad but in seeking possible sources of anxiety it is advisable to enquire into a patient's occupation (occupational stress is a common source of anxiety), family and home circumstances, social circumstances and the state of any intimate relationships.

Management

Explaining the nature of anxiety, how symptoms are generated and reassurance regarding the generally benign nature of the condition are important parts of the management of anxiety. Reducing consumption of stimulants (e.g. tea, coffee, cigarettes etc.) and reducing sources of stress are also important. More specific treatments include behavioural approaches including various forms of relaxation therapy and cognitive approaches such as problem-solving techniques and mixtures of the two such as cognitive behaviour therapy (CBT). Pharmacotherapy is not a first-line treatment for generalised anxiety disorder but it may be required in more persistent and severe cases. Among the forms of pharmacotherapy used in anxiety are anti-depressants (particularly the SSRIs and related newer anti-depressants), benzodiazepines, and beta-blockers. There are also a number of herbal remedies used by patients, usually without consultation with a doctor.

Depression

In the patient who presents with depression as a symptom it is important to distinguish between depression as used in the lay sense of the word, sometimes referred to as 'ordinary sadness' or 'life-pain', and depression amenable to medical interventions, often called 'clinical depression'. Distinguishing these is not easy and, indeed, they may be related across a spectrum of experiences of sadness or ennui, which encompasses lay notions of depression, mild, moderate and severe clinical depression. Depression, as a symptom, may also be indicative of a number of other psychiatric conditions including:

- anxiety
- adjustment disorders
- schizophrenia
- abnormal grief reaction
- seasonal affective disorder (SAD).

Diagnostic pointers

Key indicators of clinical depression include:

- persistent low mood
- early morning waking
- anhedonia (inability to enjoy anything)
- psychomotor retardation
- feelings of guilt and/or worthlessness
- despondency about the future
- suicidal ideation or intent.

It should be noted, though, that patients without many of these symptoms may be depressed and depression can manifest itself with any number of physical symptoms – of which loss of appetite, constipation, chest pain, back pain and headache are among the more common. Furthermore almost any chronic disease a patient has for a long time may

Box 4.48 Physical illnesses associated with
an increased incidence of depression

Cardiac	Congenital and acquired disorders
Respiratory	Chronic obstructive airways disease
Neurological	Multiple sclerosis, Parkinson's disease, dementia, stroke, motor neurone disease, trauma, epilepsy
Endocrine	Thyroid disorders, Cushing's disease, diabetes, Addison's disease
Metabolic	Liver and renal failure, hypercalcaemia, B12/folate-deficient anaemia
Infective	Post-influenza, brucellosis, infectious mononucleosis, hepatitis
Joint	Arthritis and other connective tissue diseases
Iatrogenic	Primarily from drugs, e.g. steroids, L-dopa, H_2 receptor blockers, anticonvulsants
Chronic pain	
Malignancy	

eventually lead to depression (see Box 4.48). Depression can also be induced by drugs and alcohol.

Management

Management has to be tailored to the needs of patient and the severity of the condition. More severe forms of depression will generally require anti-depressant medication while milder forms may not. Where suicidal ideation is a feature, referral to a psychiatrist is required. If the risk of suicide is regarded to be at all active, emergency referral is required. If an actively suicidal patient is unwilling to accept referral on a voluntary basis compulsory referral under the terms of the relevant mental health legislation must be undertaken. General counselling or supportive psychotherapy may be useful in the short-term after the patient first presents with depression. More specific forms of counselling/psychotherapy such as cognitive-behavioural therapy and interpersonal therapy have also been shown, in clinical trials, to be beneficial for depression.

Insomnia

Insomnia may be of short or long duration. Transient insomnia of a few days duration can be due to excitement or anxiety, especially related to imminent events. It passes quickly and does not require treatment. Short-term insomnia, of a few days or weeks duration, may be related to somewhat more chronic stressors but goes when the stressors diminish and, likewise, should not need treatment. Chronic insomnia, lasting 3 or more nights per week for a month or more, is more troublesome and may need treatment with a hypnotic to restore normal sleep patterns, even after the causative factor is identified and eliminated (if possible) (Box 4.49).

Diagnostic pointers

Enquiry about the patient's lifestyle may reveal factors there, while an enquiry about recent life events may also indicate the cause. The enquiry should also deal with consumption of legal and (if appropriate) illegal drugs. Alcohol induces sleep in the short term but regular use leads to disturbance of sleep patterns, while caffeine and related compounds

Box 4.49   Causes of insomnia

Likely	**Possible**
Lifestyle factors – irregular hours, shift work, sedentary occupation	Sleep apnoea
	Narcolepsy
Alcohol and drugs, including caffeine	Paroxysmal nocturnal dyspnoea (typically in left ventricular failure)
Depression	Nocturia, e.g. secondary to prostatism
Anxiety	
Stress	Hyperthyroidism
Pain	Restless leg syndrome
Nocturnal cough (typically associated with asthma)	Peripheral vascular disease
	Psychotic illness
Noise disturbance	Abnormal grief reaction
	Misuse of hypnotics or other sedative medicines

tend to keep patients awake. Depression is characterised by a pattern of insomnia in which the patient can get to sleep but, typically, wakes up in the early hours of the morning and is unable to return to sleep – referred to as 'early morning waking'. Anxiety, by contrast, more typically is associated with difficulty in getting off to sleep in the first place – so-called 'initial insomnia'. Enquiry about the patient's work, home and intimate life may reveal the most relevant likely psychosocial stressors that might be contributing to insomnia. A thorough systems review should reveal any underlying painful or other chronic health problems. Patients may also know what is keeping them awake.

Management

Management, ideally, should be tailored to the cause of the insomnia. Underlying physical or mental illness needs to be properly diagnosed and treated. Transient and short-term insomnia usually do not require specific treatment and should resolve with time. More severe short-term insomnia and chronic insomnia may need more active management, ideally, with some combination of psychotherapy and hypnotics. All patients with insomnia, and even well people who do not, can also benefit in terms of quantity and quality of their sleep by procedures collectively known as 'sleep hygiene' (Box 4.50).

137

Confusion/disorientation

Confusion is most common in the elderly and often presents as disorientation in time, place and/or person. In the elderly, chronic confusion is usually related to one or other of the various forms of dementia (which will not be detailed here). Acute confusion in a younger person is unusual but is potentially life threatening and will almost invariably require urgent referral (see Box 4.51).

Diagnostic pointers

Signs and symptoms of underlying diseases need to be very actively sought. Thus cough and temperature would suggest

Box 4.50   Outline of sleep hygiene regimen

During the evening
- Put the day to rest – think it through, tie up loose ends in your mind and plan ahead
- Try to keep fit
- Do not sleep or doze in an armchair – no naps longer than 20 minutes
- Restrict caffeine, alcohol and nicotine as these substances impair sleep

At bedtime
- Set the alarm for the same time every day, 7 days a week until a sleep pattern is established
- Do not read or watch TV in bed – keep these activities for another room
- Put the light out when you get into bed

If problems occur
- If awake for more than 20 minutes, get up and go into another room
- Do something else and remember – most people cope well even after a sleepless night
- Go back to bed when you are 'sleepy'
- A good sleep pattern may take weeks to establish, 'stick to the plan' until then

respiratory tract infection while urinalysis with signs of infection would suggest urinary tract infection. A large variety of drugs, both legal and illegal, are associated with confusion. This is particularly likely where more than the recommended amount of drug is taken or it is taken with alcohol. Stroke is usually identified by paralysis and alteration in sensation accompanying it. Hypoxia arises in situations of usually fairly obvious cardiac and/or respiratory failure. Urinary or blood testing should enable hyperglycaemia to be identified but only blood testing (with a glucometer) will reveal hypoglycaemia. Trauma will often be identified from obvious head or other injuries but needs to be considered even in the absence of obvious injury or history of injury. Alcohol withdrawal will, obviously, be associated with excessive consumption but this will not

Box 4.51 Causes of confusion in a younger person

Likely	**Possible**
Infections (respiratory and urinary infection are particularly commonly associated)	Alcohol withdrawal
	Renal failure
	Liver failure
	Hypothyroidism
Drugs – typically prescribed medicines in older patients and recreational drugs in younger patients; alcohol possible in any age group	Hyperthyroidism
	Cerebral tumour
	Cushing's disease
	Epilepsy (post-ictal state)
Stroke	
Hypoxia (respiratory and cardiac causes)	
Diabetic complication – either hypo or hyperglycaemia	
Trauma	

always be admitted by the patient. Likewise, in epilepsy there is often an antecedent history but this may not always be disclosed. Other causes will usually be uncovered during hospital investigation.

Management

The management of confusion needs to be targeted at any underlying condition. In the absence of obvious and readily treatable causes (such as a respiratory or urinary tract infection) referral to hospital will be required.

Hallucinations

Hallucinations are experiences reported by patients whereby they have had a sensory experience for which there is no apparent corresponding physical reality. Hallucinations can relate to any of the senses but are most commonly auditory (hearing things) or visual (seeing things). Causes are listed in Box 4.52.

Box 4.52   Causes of hallucinations

Likely	**Possible**
Depression	Organic brain disease (e.g.
Schizophrenia	brain tumours)
Paranoia	Epilepsy
Hallucinogenic drugs	
(ecstasy, LSD)	
Alcohol withdrawal	

Diagnostic pointers

The form and content of hallucination may provide pointers to their cause. Thus third-person auditory hallucinations in which the patient feels there are voices referring to the patient in the third person (e.g. saying the patient is a homo-sexual) are associated with schizophrenia and/or paranoia. By contrast second-person hallucinations (e.g. 'you are worthless') are less likely to be associated with schizophre-nia and their content (e.g. if it is derogatory) may point to a particular diagnosis such as depression. Alcohol withdrawal may be associated with particularly vivid hallucinations which may be multimodal i.e. auditory and tactile. Visual hallucinations, in particular, are more likely in organic brain disorders but less common types of hallucination, e.g. olfactory hallucinations, may also be indicative of epilepsy or other organic causes.

Management

The underlying cause of hallucinations, if it can be identi-fied, should be treated as a priority. Some symptom relief will usually be provided by major tranquillisers such as the phenothiazines. Hallucinations are manifestations of more serious mental illness and patients displaying them should be referred to a specialist psychiatrist.

Delusions

A delusion is a fixed firm belief that is not affected by rational argument or contrary evidence and is not conven-

140

Box 4.53   Causes of delusions

Likely	**Possible**
Depression	Hypochondriasis (content
Schizophrenia	concerned with illness)
Paranoia (content usually	Folie-a-deux
paranoid)	Alcoholism

tional given the patient's cultural background. Thus, believing in God is not considered a delusion but believing firmly that you are God is. Causes are listed in Box 4.53.

Diagnostic pointers

As with hallucinations, the nature and content of the delusion may give an indication of its cause. Delusions of guilt and worthlessness and other nihilistic-type delusions are typically associated with depression. Persecutory delusions and delusions of reference are typically associated with paranoia. Delusions of grandeur and delusions of control (e.g. thought control) are typically associated with schizophrenia, although delusions of all types can occur in this condition. Delusions of jealously are associated with alcoholism in men.

141

Management

Delusions are indicators of severe mental illness and patients with delusions would usually be referred to psychiatrists.

Further Reading

Ballinger A, Patchett S 2003 Saunders' pocket essentials of clinical medicine, 3rd edn. W B Saunders, Edinburgh

Buxton P K 2003 ABC of dermatology, 4th edn. BMJ Books, London

Cartwright S, Goodlee C 2003 Churchill's pocketbook of general practice, 2nd edn. Churchill Livingstone, Edinburgh

Hopcroft K, Forte V 2003 Symptom sorter, 2nd edn. Radcliffe Medical Press, Oxford

Khot A, Polmear A 2003 Practical general practice, 4th edn. Butterworth Heinemann, Edinburgh

Kumar P, Clark M 2002 Clinical medicine, 5th edn. W B Saunders, Edinburgh

Murtagh J 2003 General practice, 3rd edn. McGraw Hill, New York

Smith D S 1999 Field guide to bedside diagnosis. Lippincott Williams & Wilkins, New York

Chronic Illness

Importance in general practice

Chronic diseases are now among the commonest causes of death in most industrialised and many developing countries. People who in the past would have succumbed to acute medical problems now survive, frequently due to medical intervention, to live for many years. However, they are often living with the burden of chronic sequelae of acute illnesses. Furthermore, due to improvements in general health many people now live long enough to acquire one or more chronic, usually degenerative, disease(s).

Other trends in health service development, such as the preference for healthcare funding agencies to shift care from hospitals to the community, mean that the management of chronic disease comprises an ever-increasing proportion of GPs' workload. Thus, not only are GPs looking after more and more people with chronic diseases, they are also expected to provide a greater proportion of their care.

All this requires GPs to be better trained, better equipped, better organised and better resourced. With increasingly serious chronic illnesses, the quality of care provided becomes more critical to the outcome for the patient. The outcome in acute life-threatening emergencies presenting in primary care is substantially determined by speed of transfer to and the quality of secondary care. However, the outcome for a patient with chronic illness is critically dependent on GP input.

If a patient with asthma has a GP who does not have a systematic approach to providing education about the condition and its care, the patient may drift from asthma attack to asthma attack without ever receiving an adequate understanding of the condition and its treatment. A patient whose GP embarks on systematic education about asthma and regularly monitors peak flows, symptoms and response to treatment, is likely to suffer fewer attacks and fewer hospital admissions. It could be said that having a well organised and effective GP can make the difference between *having* a chronic disease and *suffering* from it.

Effective management

Effective management of any chronic disease is designed to reduce the risk of exacerbations or complications of the disease, or both. It necessitates monitoring indicators (such as symptoms and/or biological parameters), prescribing and monitoring treatment, and educating the patient about the disease and its treatment.

To be effective in this role the GP needs a well organised practice with good information and administration systems, including a systematic approach dictating what checks will be done and at what frequency. It will also usually involve having a system to call or recall patients, particularly those who fail to attend. To deliver high-quality care requires a good knowledge and understanding of all aspects of the disease in question, including its pathogenesis, clinical manifestations and management. The competent GP will know what treatments are available, how these need to be dispensed and monitored, and what complications or other facets of the disease need to be ascertained and followed.

To engage the patient constructively and effectively in the management of any condition requires good rapport and relationship-building skills (see Chapter 9). The GP also needs to be a good educator – this requires leadership qualities and enthusiasm.

Chronic disease management is about doing the little things well, which is not as easy as it sounds. A key to maintaining quality of chronic disease care is to regularly review your performance against some externally validated standard. This process is often referred to as medical or clinical 'audit'. The process of performance review is now becoming an integral part of re-accreditation and is being written into GP contracts as so-called 'quality indicators'. See Box 5.1 for an outline of effective management.

Role of the GP

The initial diagnosis may be made by the GP or by a hospital specialist, or be confirmed by the hospital specialist at the GP's request. The specialist making or confirming the diagnosis will often devise the initial management plan, though this may need to be further refined and modified by the GP to better suit the particular patient (Box 5.2). For some chronic illnesses diagnosis and management is handled entirely by the GP.

Box 5.1   Effective management of chronic disease

- Well organised practice:
  - good information systems
  - systematic approach
  - call and recall systems for defaulters
- Good knowledge and understanding of the disease including:
  - pathogenesis
  - symptoms
  - signs
  - complications
  - treatments available
- Monitoring of appropriate clinical and laboratory indicators
- Good rapport and relationship-building skills
- Active engagement of patients in the management of their own conditions
- Education of patients
- Regular reviews (audits) of quality of care against some external standard

Regardless of who devises the management plan it will ultimately be implemented by the patient, supported by the GP. The GP will usually need to recruit the assistance of other primary healthcare team members (see Chapter 10). For common and important chronic diseases the GP will need to set up information systems to register and monitor the progress of all practice patients with each condition.

A system to call and recall patients may also be required, as patients with a chronic disease may forget their treatment, or certain aspects of it, if not regularly reminded. They may also be deteriorating or developing complications of which they are not aware.

A guideline or protocol determining the content and procedures to be followed at each patient visit should be devised, ideally in collaboration with the hospital specialist and/or with the primary healthcare team. Indeed, guidelines are increasingly being written into the contractual arrangements between GPs and their employers.

GPs need to explore all facets of the patient's illness – including physical, psychological, and social aspects. The

GP has a major role in assisting the patient get any appropriate and necessary services from other sources, including hospitals and other agencies, and from voluntary and self-help groups. In this role the GP is often acting as a patient advocate (see Box 5.2).

In many instances to carry out these functions effectively the GP will need to set aside time exclusively to a particular chronic problem in the form of a chronic disease management clinic. Such clinics will usually be run jointly between the GP and a nurse – and other primary healthcare team members as appropriate. A list of parameters to be checked at each visit should be specified in a guideline or protocol for the management of the disease.

There should also be an education programme about the disease and its management, which is provided to each patient – usually over a series of clinic visits. This programme should encourage and enable the patient to manage the condition as much as possible. As a minimum, each patient will be expected to adhere to any agreed management plan, including taking any necessary medicines. It is also helpful if the GP is aware of and can recommend any self-help or patient groups who will be able to provide the

Box 5.2 The role of the GP

- Make/confirm the diagnosis (sometimes)
- Devise a management plan or refine the hospital management plan, if required
- With the patient, implement the management plan
- Recruit assistance and support of other primary healthcare team(s)
- Monitor progress of disease and effects of treatment
- Attend to all aspects of the illness (physical, psychological and social)
- Devise and follow the guideline or protocol for each patient visit
- Act as a patient advocate
- Education of patients
- Inform patients about self-help groups

patient with additional information and support in looking after each condition.

Role of guidelines

To ensure the highest standards of care for patients with chronic diseases, it is important that what is done for them is not left to the vagaries of what different doctors think is the right thing to do. Guidelines should be based on research evidence as to what works. As the techniques of evidence-based medicine have been refined and developed, guidelines increasingly come complete with a gradation of the quality of evidence on which they are based and with references to the relevant evidence base.

As research continues and the evidence base improves it is important that guidelines are updated, so guidelines should also come with an expiry date. Comprehensive sets of guidelines following these principals have now been collated and developed by the Scottish Intercollegiate Guidelines Network (SIGN – www.sign.ac.uk) (NICE – www.nice.org.uk) and in Scandinavia by Duodecim (www.ebm-guidelines.com).

Once a set of guidelines has been provided active steps need to be taken to ensure that they are disseminated to practising clinicians. It has also been shown that guidelines will be implemented more effectively if those who are applying them feel some sense of ownership. This can be done by allowing discussion of the guidelines before adoption and, ideally, giving them some degree of local 'spin' – such as tailoring them to a particular practice's existing healthcare partners.

The implementation of guidelines is also reinforced if the care delivered is subjected to a process of regular performance review or audit.

Performance review

If we collect data on the care actually received by our patients and compare it to the care we intended to give them, we can see that we often fail to do quite what we

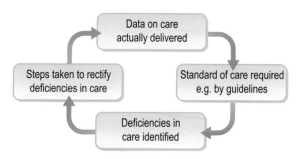

Fig. 5.1 **The audit cycle**

intended. The mere act of collecting and looking at such data is a powerful stimulus to improving performance.

This systematic comparison of the care actually delivered with care that is intended to be delivered, with a view to improving the standard of that care, is referred to in the UK as 'medical audit'. A somewhat broader term of 'clinical audit' is applied when the process involves healthcare workers other than doctors. In other places the process is referred to as performance review. It is important to realise that the process should be a continuous one, resonating, as it does, with the notions of 'continuous quality improvement' and 'total quality management'. It is sometimes described as the quality cycle (Fig. 5.1), whereby data on care delivered is collected, compared to a standard (such as expert evidence-based guidelines, see above), deficiencies noted and decisions made on how to address them, followed by a review at a later date to see if matters have improved.

149

Specific chronic conditions

Diabetes mellitus

Essential background information

Diabetes is a metabolic disorder characterised by raised blood glucose. There are two main types:

- Type 1 diabetes is characterised by a total lack of endogenous insulin.
- Type 2 diabetes is associated with progressive pancreatic beta-cell failure and hence inadequate beta-cell secretion of insulin, although there are also associated problems with insulin action at end-organs (i.e. insulin resistance).

Type 1 diabetes occurs at all ages and must be treated with insulin. Type 2 diabetes typically occurs later in life (over 40) and is associated with obesity. The overall prevalence of diabetes is about 2%, of which over 80% of cases are type 2 diabetes. Patients with type 1 diabetes are susceptible to diabetic ketoacidosis which, if untreated, can lead to coma and death. Once on treatment they may also be susceptible to hypoglycaemia, which may also lead to coma and death if unrecognised and untreated. Both types of diabetes are prone to longer-term complications, most of which are associated with either micro- or macrovascular disease related to raised blood glucose.

According to WHO criteria, fasting plasma glucose of over 7.0 mmol/L is diagnostic of diabetes, as is a random or 2-hour post-glucose load level of 11.1 mmol/L or more. Because of the seriousness of a diagnosis of diabetes, two tests with these levels are required before a diagnosis is made. Patients with fasting plasma glucose of 6.1–6.9 mmol/L and 2-hour post glucose load level of <7.8 mmol/L are defined as having 'impaired fasting glycaemia'. Those with a fasting plasma glucose level <7.0 mmol/L and a 2-hour post glucose load plasma glucose of 7.8–11.0 mmol/L are defined as having 'impaired glucose tolerance' – the implication being that patients with these conditions are at increased risk of both diabetes and heart disease.

Clinical features

Type 1 initial presentation

The classic symptoms of type 1 diabetes at presentation are polyuria, polydipsia, and weight loss which are usually of a relatively short duration (i.e. a few days to a few weeks).

Patients may also present acutely unwell with manifestations of ketoacidosis such as lethargy, altered level of consciousness, hyperventilation and breath that smells of ketones (the smell of ketones is similar to that of nail varnish remover, which contains acetone, a basic ketone).

Type 2 initial presentation

Initial presentation of type 2 diabetes is usually more insidious and may be with complications of the disease rather than primary manifestations of raised glucose per se. Thus patients with type 2 diabetes may first present diabetic complications such as Candida infection, a neuropathy, renal or eye disease, or with a cardiovascular event.

Management of diabetes

Type 1 diabetes

Type 1 diabetes requires treatment with insulin injections – usually multiple injections per day – comprising a mixture of long-action and rapid-acting forms of insulin. Type 1 diabetes is usually managed by a specialist with input from the GP. Assiduous attention to diet and physical activity levels are required in order to maintain blood glucose levels within the desired range of 4.4–6.1 mmol/L. Glucose levels can usually be measured by the patient using a blood glucose monitor. Research has shown that maintaining tight control is associated with a reduced risk of complications, although if control is too tight the patient may suffer severe episodes of hypoglycaemia. A key to good glucose control is good patient education (see below).

Type 2 diabetes

First-line treatment of type 2 diabetes comprises modifications to lifestyle, particularly diet. The recommended diet is essentially the same as that recommended to the general population for good health i.e. low in fat (no more than 30% of energy intake and primarily unsaturated fats), low in simple carbohydrates (such as sugar) but with 50–55% of energy intake in the form of complex carbohydrates and 15% of energy intake in the form of protein.

However, patients with diabetes have to be more meticulous about their diet and need to particularly avoid foods with a high glycaemic index. Glycaemic index is an indicator of the amount of glucose released shortly after ingestion of a food. Simple carbohydrates tend to have higher glycaemic indices than complex carbohydrates and foods with a lower glycaemic index tend to aid metabolic control in diabetes. The nutrient load from foods should be spread throughout the day and calorie intake should be appropriate to the patient's age, gender and levels of physical activity.

Physical activity levels should be increased, alcohol intake should be restricted to recommended maximum levels (i.e. 21 units/week for men and 14 units/week for women) and patients who smoke should be helped to quit.

Where lifestyle modification fails to bring glucose levels down to the required levels a drug treatment may be required. The principal types of oral anti-diabetic agent are biguanides and sulphonylureas, although there are several new agents also available whose place in therapy is not yet clearly established.

The care of patients with type 2 diabetes is increasingly shared between GPs and specialists in various integrated or shared-care schemes. A small proportion of patients with type 2 diabetes may receive all their care from the GP and primary healthcare team.

Drugs used in management

Biguanides

The only available biguanide is metformin (see the British National Formulary for dosages). It exerts its effect mainly by decreasing gluconeogenesis and by increasing peripheral utilisation of glucose. It is particularly useful in obese patients as it is associated with less weight gain than sulphonylureas. It is also less likely to cause hypoglycaemia. It may also be used in conjunction with a sulphonylurea to improve blood glucose control. However, it may cause gastrointestinal disturbances, especially when first used.

Sulphonylureas

These act mainly by increasing insulin production by pancreatic beta cells. In overdose they can cause hypoglycaemia. They may also encourage weight gain and are best avoided in obese patients, except, perhaps, in combination with metformin. Adverse effects, particularly hypoglycaemia, are more frequent with longer-acting sulphonylureas (such as chlorpropamide and glibenclamide) and in the elderly – especially with renal or hepatic impairment. Shorter-acting sulphonylureas such as gliclazide and tolbutamide are generally to be preferred for such patients.

Acarbose

Acarbose acts by inhibiting gastrointestinal enzymes, thereby delaying and reducing intestinal absorption of sucrose and starches. It is generally used in conjunction with metformin or a sulphonylurea. Flatulence is the main side effect.

Nateglinide and repaglinide

These are newer agents that also act to increase insulin release. They are rapid acting with a short duration of action and so can be used after meals to simulate normal insulin. Repaglinide may be used as monotherapy or with metformin but nateglinide is licensed for use only with metformin.

Pioglitazone and rosiglitazone ('glitazones')

These act by reducing peripheral insulin resistance. They are used exclusively in combination with either metformin or a sulphonylurea, but not both. They may cause liver dysfunction – patients on these agents must have their liver function monitored after starting treatment.

Insulin therapy in type 2 diabetes

As beta-cell function continues to deteriorate, blood glucose control may become more difficult to achieve and a proportion of patients with type 2 diabetes will require treatment with insulin. The switch to insulin treatment is often resisted by the patient and by doctors but this is preferable to neglecting poor control, thereby increasing the risk of complications. A changeover to insulin therapy is often associated with an undesirable weight gain. This problem can be minimised by close attention to diet and physical activity levels at the time of the changeover. The move to insulin therapy is frequently managed in secondary care but as primary care of diabetes improves this transition is coming to be managed more often in the community.

Management of other risk factors

While the management of diabetes is very much focused on blood glucose control, it must also be remembered that diabetes is a major risk factor for cardiovascular disease and so other aspects of cardiovascular disease risk need close attention too. Patients with diabetes should control their body weight with diet and exercise such that their body mass index is maintained within the normal range (BMI 20–25). They should also be strongly urged to give up smoking if they smoke and supported in efforts to cease smoking with nicotine replacement treatment or bupropion as appropriate.

Blood pressure should be tightly controlled with the recommended target level being below 130/85 mmHg. Likewise, LDL cholesterol should be kept below 2.6 mmol/L. There is also good evidence to support an approach to cardiovascular risk management in diabetes similar to that advocated for secondary prevention of cardiovascular disease (see below) in patients who have already suffered an event. Thus, treatment with ACE inhibitors (which have an additional reno-protective effect), beta-blockers, aspirin, and statins must all be considered.

Complications

Important long-term complications include:

- diabetic eye disease
- diabetic nephropathy

- diabetic neuropathy
- cardiovascular disease – now recognised as the major cause of morbidity and mortality in patients with diabetes.

Diabetic eye disease

Diabetes is associated with a number of ocular complications. These include:

- diabetic retinopathy (the commonest)
- diabetic maculopathy
- cataracts
- glaucoma
- ocular palsies.

Diabetic retinopathy begins with the development of capillary microaneurysms and leakage of fluids from retinal capillaries. These appear as dot haemorrhages and exudates on examination of the fundi. Later, new vessels begin to appear (neovascularisation) – at which stage it is referred to as proliferative retinopathy. This can be treated with laser photocoagulation if caught early enough. It is now possible to detect early signs of proliferative retinopathy using retinal photography, which is increasingly being used to monitor patients with diabetes for eye disease. Patients with diabetes need regular ophthalmic examinations but where access to an ophthalmologist is restricted retinal photography offers a potential solution to the need to screen all patients with diabetes at regular (annual) intervals.

Diabetic nephropathy

Sustained hyperglycaemia leads to renal disease, mainly through actions on the glomerulus. The earliest observable indication of renal damage is 'microalbuminuria' – an increase in urinary albumin above the normal range. If detected, diabetic nephropathy is first managed by tight blood pressure control with an ACE inhibitor.

Diabetic neuropathy

Diabetes may be associated with both somatic and autonomic neuropathies. Somatic neuropathies are typically symmetrical and affect sensory nerves. Other somatic neuropathies include painful neuropathies of single nerves, mononeuropathies of cranial (especially III and VI) or other motor nerves, and amyotrophies (especially affecting the quadriceps). Peripheral neuropathies are particularly associated with the development of 'diabetic foot' where, partly due to loss of sensation, but possibly compounded by macrovascular and microvascular disease, one or both feet develop one or more of a variety of problems. The most significant of these problems is tissue necrosis, which may lead to ulcers and possibly even amputation if not adequately treated. Treatment involves wound care including debridement if needed, close monitoring of peripheral blood supply, e.g. by Doppler, and vascular surgery if necessary. Autonomic neuropathy can present with postural hypotension, gustatory sweating, gastroparesis, erectile dysfunction (impotence), diarrhoea or urinary incontinence.

Monitoring

In view of all the possible complications of diabetes and its strong association with the development of ischaemic heart disease there are a large number of parameters that need to be monitored, including:

- blood glucose – home readings, clinic readings (fasting or random)
- HbA1 or fructosamine
- urine for microalbuminuria
- body mass index
- blood pressure
- fundoscopy – with dilated pupils
- feet for redness, abrasions, callosities, evidence of impaired circulation (especially diminished pulses)
- adherence to diet and/or medications.

Primary healthcare team members

The primary care team members to involve will include, in varying roles and functions depending on the patient:

- DM 3. The percentage of patients with diabetes in whom there is a record of smoking status in the previous 15 months, except those who have never smoked where smoking status should be recorded once
- DM 4. The percentage of patients with diabetes who smoke and whose notes contain a record that smoking cessation advice has been offered in the last 15 months
- DM 5. The percentage of diabetic patients who have a record of HbA1c or equivalent in the previous 15 months
- DM 6. The percentage of patients with diabetes in whom the last HbA1c is 7.4 or less (or equivalent test/reference range depending on local laboratory) in last 15 months
- DM 7. The percentage of patients with diabetes in whom the last HbA1c is 10 or less (or equivalent test/reference range depending on local laboratory) in last 15 months
- DM 8. The percentage of patients with diabetes who have a record of retinal screening in the previous 15 months
- DM 9. The percentage of patients with diabetes with a record of presence or absence of peripheral pulses in the previous 15 months
- DM 10. The percentage of patients with diabetes with a record of neuropathy testing in the previous 15 months
- DM 11. The percentage of patients with diabetes who have a record of the blood pressure in the past 15 months
- DM 12. The percentage of patients with diabetes in whom the last blood pressure is 145/85 or less
- DM 13. The percentage of patients with diabetes who have a record of microalbuminuria testing in the previous 15 months (exception reporting for patients with proteinuria)
- DM 14. The percentage of patients with diabetes who have a record of serum creatinine testing in the previous 15 months
- DM 15. The percentage of patients with diabetes with proteinuria or microalbuminuria who are treated with ACE inhibitors (or A2 antagonists)
- DM 16. The percentage of patients with diabetes who have a record of total cholesterol in the previous 15 months
- DM 17. The percentage of patients with diabetes whose last measured total cholesterol within previous 15 months is 5 or less
- DM 18. The percentage of patients with diabetes who have had influenza immunisation in the preceding 1 September to 31 March

modifiable – modification of such risk factors has been shown to reduce risks of developing manifestations of the disease.

Definitions/diagnosis

Angina pectoris

While, strictly speaking, the term 'angina pectoris' refers to the characteristic pain in the chest associated with ischaemic heart disease, the use of the word 'angina' has become generalised to include all manifestations of impaired perfusion of coronary vessels up to but excluding myocardial infarction. Typically it is associated with a discomfort or pain in the centre of the chest, which may radiate to the left neck, jaw, shoulder or arm and may be induced by physical and/or emotional exertion. The pain may be relieved by rest and by nitrates.

Cardiac failure

As the term 'cardiac failure' suggests, this is a condition associated with failure of the heart to fulfil its functions. However, there are many different causes and manifestations of varying extents and degrees of cardiac failure. Heart failure is often classified into right and left heart failure on the basis of clinical manifestations, with right heart failure being associated with systemic venous congestion (oedema, raised jugular venous pulse etc.) and left heart failure being associated with pulmonary venous congestion (e.g. dyspnoea, basal crackles).

Acute myocardial infarction

Acute myocardial infarction occurs when there is sudden and complete obstruction of blood flow to one or more coronary arteries and resultant death or infarction of myocardial muscle. The abrupt loss of myocardium (and hence the heart's pump function) and/or associated arrhythmias means that acute myocardial infarction is often fatal. When it occurs it constitutes a medical emergency (see Chapter 3).

Angina pectoris

Clinical features

The typical pain of angina is a precordial pain, sometimes perceived more as a discomfort or feeling of pressure, which is brought on by physical exertion and relieved by rest. It can also be induced by emotional upset or it may come on after a large meal. It is also usually relieved by nitrate medications that can be taken immediately as sublingual nitroglycerine tablets or spray. During attacks pulse rate and blood pressure may become elevated but often, especially between attacks, there may be no abnormal signs at all.

Angina occurring at rest or at night is more ominous as it usually indicates a more severe degree of coronary artery occlusion. Angina that is coming in more frequent and severe attacks, known as 'crescendo angina', may be indicative of an impending myocardial infarction. Indeed, any irregularity in the pattern of angina attacks may be indicative of more severe ischaemic heart disease. Variant or Prinzmetal angina is a form of angina with a range of severe symptoms sometimes associated with arrhythmia and with ECG changes (of ST elevation) during attacks. It is associated with spasm of coronary arteries close to major obstructions. There is also a condition referred to as 'syndrome X', in which patients who have radiographically normal coronary arteries have symptoms typical of angina.

Management

There are two main goals in the management of angina. The first is to relieve the symptoms of angina and the second is to reduce the risk of a myocardial infarction or other cardiovascular event.

Nitrates

These are given as sublingual tablets or spray for immediate relief of symptoms or as long-acting oral preparations or in the form of nitrate patches. Tolerance can build up if nitrates are given continuously and so nitrate-free intervals must be included in the regimen. Headache, palpitation and dizziness – all related to the vasodilator effects of nitrates – are the commoner side effects.

Beta-blockers

There are many different beta-blockers, all of which relieve angina, but the so-called 'cardioselective' beta-blockers such as atenolol are said to have a lower risk of inducing bronchospasm. Beta-blockers may have additional advantages of reducing blood pressure and are also known to reduce the risk of myocardial infarction, especially in patients who have already had an MI. However, they can exacerbate heart failure through a negative inotropic effect and they can worsen peripheral vascular disease.

Dihydropyridine calcium antagonists

Dihydropyridine calcium channel blockers (e.g. nifedipine and amlodipine) have vasodilating effects on coronary arteries and can be useful in reducing angina symptoms. They also reduce blood pressure and coronary artery spasm. Other calcium channel blockers also reduce angina symptoms, e.g. by direct effects on cardiac muscle, but negative intropic effects may render them less ideal choices. Adverse effects include headache, flushing and ankle swelling, which are related to vasodilatation, and sinus bradycardia and/or heart block, which may be related to negative intropic effects.

Nicorandil

This is a relatively new anti-anginal drug used where other treatments are incompletely effective. It has vasodilating effects on both coronary and peripheral arteries and it is also venodilating. Thus it is believed to reduce cardiac pre-load and after-load and relieves coronary artery spasm. It has all the vasodilator side effects of nitrates and calcium channel blockers and is contraindicated in heart failure and hypotension.

Surgical interventions

As well as drug treatments, angina may also be relieved by coronary revascularisation procedures such as coronary artery bypass and transcutaneous coronary angioplasty with or without insertion of a stent in appropriate patients – i.e. patients with well-localised disease as determined on angiography and severe or unstable or medically unresponsive angina. In view of the potential benefits of revascularisation procedures it is important that all patients with angina be fully evaluated with exercise stress-testing, followed by angiography if the stress test is positive for probable IHD.

Management of cardiovascular risk factors is discussed in Chapter 6.

Monitoring

Patients should be monitored at regular intervals to ensure that they are receiving adequate symptom relief from their treatment. They should also be monitored to ensure they are in receipt of all appropriate measures to reduce cardiovascular risk including smoking cessation advice, support and treatment (if required), anti-hypertensive treatment (if required), lipid-lowering drugs (if required), dietary advice and support, an exercise programme and aspirin (if the individual patient can tolerate it).

What the patient should know

The patient with angina should know that they have ischaemic heart disease and that it is a long-term condition for which there is no cure but which can, with appropriate medicines and lifestyle modification, be controlled. They need to try and avoid obvious precipitants of symptoms such as severe exertion but they should not be allowed to become so obsessive about avoiding symptoms that they severely limit their daily lives or unnecessarily impair its quality. Moderate exercise is manageable by most patients and normal sexual activity does not usually need to be limited. Patients probably ought to be warned that they do have an increased risk of myocardial infarction and, indeed, other cardiovascular disease and may have a reduced life expectancy – although this information ought to be given in the more encouraging context that lifestyle modifications and other risk-reduction strategies are effective in minimising these risks.

What should be checked in a performance review

A practice register of patients with ischaemic heart disease should be available. This should indicate the type of IHD and the patient's risk profile, listing the parameters in Box 5.5. Actions to reduce risks should also be recorded and the proportion of patients in receipt of these should be reviewed (Box 5.6).

For angina patients there should be a record of the proportion of patients who have had exercise-stress test or other specialist assessment and a record of the proportion of patients whose medical therapy is controlling their symptoms. See Box 5.7 for the contractually required measures.

Box 5.5   Patient's risk profile for angina pectoris

- Smoking status (i.e. smoker, non-smoker, or ex-smoker; number of cigarettes per day smoked and for how many years etc.)
- Blood pressure
- Body mass index
- Fasting cholesterol level (or lipid profile)
- Family history of IHD in first-degree relatives
- Diabetes if present
- Usual level of physical activity

Box 5.6   Actions taken to reduce risk

- Smoking cessation
- Dietary advice
- Exercise programmes
- Antihypertensive drugs
- Lipid-lowering drugs (especially statins)
- Aspirin therapy
- Influenza vaccination

Box 5.7 New GP (UK) contract requirements/
indicators for coronary heart disease

- CHD 1. The practice can produce a register of patients
  with coronary heart disease
- CHD 2. The percentage of patients with newly diagnosed
  angina (diagnosed after 01/04/03) who are referred for
  exercise testing and/or specialist assessment
- CHD 3. The percentage of patients with coronary heart
  disease, whose notes record smoking status in the past
  15 months, except those who have never smoked where
  smoking status need be recorded only once
- CHD 4. The percentage of patients with coronary heart
  disease who smoke, whose notes contain a record that
  smoking cessation advice has been offered within the last
  15 months
- CHD 5. The percentage of patients with coronary heart
  disease whose notes have a record of blood pressure in
  the previous 15 months
- CHD 6. The percentage of patients with coronary heart
  disease, in whom the last blood pressure reading
  (measured in the last 15 months) is 150/90 or less
- CHD 7. The percentage of patients with coronary heart
  disease whose notes have a record of total cholesterol in
  the previous 15 months
- CHD 8. The percentage of patients with coronary heart
  disease whose last measured total cholesterol (measured
  in the last 15 months) is 5 mmol/L or less
- CHD 9. The percentage of patients with coronary heart
  disease with a record in the last 15 months that aspirin, an
  alternative anti-platelet therapy, or an anti-coagulant is
  being taken (unless a contraindication or side effects are
  recorded)
- CHD 10. The percentage of patients with coronary heart
  disease who are currently treated with a beta-blocker
  (unless a contraindication or side effects are recorded)
- CHD 11. The percentage of patients with a history of
  myocardial infarction (diagnosed after 1 April 2003) who
  are currently treated with an ACE inhibitor
- CHD 12. The percentage of patients with coronary heart
  disease who have a record of influenza vaccination in the
  preceding 1 September to 31 March

Cardiac failure

Clinical features

The presenting features of cardiac failure will depend on whether it is principally right or left heart failure, although both sets of features may occur in combined right and left heart failure – sometimes referred to as 'congestive cardiac failure'. There are several pathophysiological mechanisms that may contribute to heart failure, each contributing to the array of clinical features present in any one case.

Increased venous pressure (related to cardiac pre-load) gives rise to cough, breathlessness, wheeze and signs of pulmonary oedema when it applies to the left ventricle and to peripheral oedema, raised jugular venous pulse and hepatomegaly when it applies to the right ventricle. Reduced cardiac output (related to cardiac after-load) gives rise to generalised fatigue, dizziness, confusion, syncope (related to impaired cerebral circulation), reduced blood pressure and tachycardia. Impairment of the cardiac pumping mechanism gives rise to ventricular dilatation, cardiomegaly, cardiac murmurs (typically a pansystolic murmur) and a gallop rhythm due to audible third and/or fourth heart sounds.

Management

Non-drug treatments include dietary measures and rest. Dietary measures include restriction of salt and sugar and reduction in overall calories to reduce body mass (obesity being a common accompaniment of cardiac failure). In acute heart failure bed rest is generally desirable but in stable chronic heart failure patients are better to stay active within the limits imposed by their disease. The usual measures to reduce cardiovascular risk (such as stopping smoking) should also be advised.

Drug treatments include diuretics, ACE inhibitors, angiotensin receptor antagonists (also known as A2 blockers), spironoluctone, certain beta-blockers and digoxin (specifically where heart failure is associated with atrial fibrillation). Cardiac transplantation is also a definitive treatment in appropriate patients.

Monitoring

Patients with heart failure need to be monitored to ensure the condition is kept under control. Echocardiogram is the best test for diagnosis and assessment of heart failure. For patients with left heart failure, symptoms such as dyspnoea on exertion may be indicators of incompletely controlled failure – as would the appearance or reappearance of basal crepitations on lung auscultation. For patients with right heart failure recurrence of typical symptoms or signs would, likewise, indicate inadequacy of control. Body weight is a particularly useful and sensitive indicator as it will increase if there is venous congestion and it ought to stabilise or be decreasing if the patient is adherent to the recommended diet. Patients on diuretics and/or ACE inhibitors/A2 blockers (which would include virtually all heart failure patients) need to have their potassium levels and renal function checked at regular intervals. Compliance with any prescribed medications and with lifestyle modification should also be reviewed regularly.

What the patient should know

The patient with heart failure needs to understand something of the nature of their condition and to know what symptoms might indicate deterioration. They need to understand the importance of adherence to advised drug and non-drug treatment in order to maximise the prognosis. Patients probably ought to be told that heart failure is a life-limiting condition which might well continue to deteriorate in spite of the GP's best therapeutic endeavours – but they should also be reassured that modern treatments, especially ACE inhibitors and A2 blockers, are known to improve their prognosis.

What should be checked in a performance review

A review of cardiac failure patients should determine the proportion on optimal drug therapy, which should include either an ACE inhibitor or an A2 blocker. The proportion of patients who have had their potassium level and renal function checked in the previous year should also be determined. The proportion of patients with various other risk factors for cardiovascular disease also ought to be checked – see above and Box 5.8.

Acute myocardial infarction

Acute myocardial infarction is dealt with in Chapter 3.

Essential hypertension

Essential background information

There are many possible causes of raised blood pressure or hypertension. However, from a general practice point of view so-called secondary hypertension – hypertension secondary to another condition such as phaeochromocytoma – is quite rare. The overwhelming majority of cases of hypertension in general practice have no identifiable primary cause – a condition called essential hypertension.

Hypertension is the commonest chronic condition treated in general practice. It is, strictly speaking, not a disease but rather it is a risk factor that predicts the probability of suffering from other diseases – specifically ischaemic heart disease and cerebrovascular disease. However, what makes

168

Box 5.8 New GP (UK) contract requirements/ indicators for left ventricular dysfunction

- LVD 1. The practice can produce a register of patients with CHD and left ventricular dysfunction
- LVD 2. The percentage of patients with a diagnosis of CHD and left ventricular dysfunction that has been confirmed by an echocardiogram
- LVD 3. The percentage of patients with a diagnosis of CHD and left ventricular dysfunction who are currently treated with ACE inhibitors (or A2 antagonists)

it seem like a disease is that it can be diagnosed and treated and, although treatment is aimed at controlling blood pressure within a target range, the principal benefit of treatment is a reduction in the risk of suffering from other conditions.

Diagnosis/definition

While there are several different definitions of hypertension in use those most commonly applied in medical practice in the UK are those proposed by the British Hypertension Society (Table 5.1). These values are based on blood pressure as measured in the routine manner in general practice or outpatient clinics. Blood pressures are increasingly measured by patients at home using electronic blood pressure monitors (home blood pressure monitoring) and ambulatory blood pressure monitors. Values obtained by these methods are typically lower than those obtained in clinic settings – due to a phenomenon known as 'the white coat effect'. Thresholds for diagnosis and treatment are lowered accordingly, but details on these adjustments are beyond the scope of this book.

169

Table 5.1
British Hypertension Society's classification of hypertension

Category	Systolic blood pressure (mmHg)	Diastolic blood pressure (mmHg)
Blood pressure		
Optimal	<120	<80
Normal	<130	<85
High normal	130–139	85–90
Hypertension		
Grade 1 (mild)	140–149	90–99
Grade 2 (moderate)	160–179	100–109
Grade 3 (severe)	≥180	≥110
Isolated systolic hypertension		
Grade 1	140–159	<90
Grade 2	≥160	<90

Clinical features

Patients with high blood pressure do not usually have any symptoms on presentation, although once informed of the diagnosis patients often will report symptoms they associate with high blood pressure such as headaches. Rarely patients with very high blood pressure, particularly malignant hypertension, may present with headaches, visual disturbance and possibly other neurological manifestations. Thus hypertension is typically diagnosed incidentally when the patient presents for other reasons or during the course of a routine health check. Although a single high blood pressure reading is associated, epidemiologically, with an increased risk of premature mortality, a decision to commence treatment is not justifiable on a single elevated reading. Three readings are usually advised before a decision is made to treat an elevated blood pressure.

Although high blood pressure does not usually present with symptoms, evidence can sometimes be found at the time of presentation of damage thought to be due to high blood pressure – this is referred to as 'end organ damage'. The heart, the kidneys and the eyes are the main organs to exhibit such end organ damage. In the heart the typical feature of end organ damage is left ventricular hypertrophy. In more severe untreated hypertension cardiac failure may also occur. Hypertension-related renal damage may be manifest with detection of protein in the urine (proteinuria) but, if severe, may progress to raised creatinine levels and other features of renal failure. In the eyes one may get hypertensive retinopathy. This, too, is a progressive condition. Early signs are narrowing of retinal arteries and so called 'silver wiring' – this progresses to signs seen at arterial intersections. Later, haemorrhages and exudates may appear and, finally, papilloedema.

Management

The aim of treatment is to reduce blood pressure to within a target range. The target to be achieved depends on other risk factors in the patient. Targets for patients in relation to their risk suggested by the British Hypertension Society are that a patient without clinically associated conditions or end organ damage can be treated to achieve a target of 140 mmHg systolic and diastolic of 90 mmHg. For patients with diabetes or established renal or cardiovascular disease the target should be set at 130 mmHg systolic and a diastolic of 80.

Non-pharmacological management

- Diet – low salt (<100 mmol/day), 5 portions per day of fruit or vegetables, reduce intake of total fat (particularly saturated fat)
- Physical activity – >30 minutes aerobic exercise most days of the week
- Cessation of tobacco consumption
- Moderation of alcohol consumption to less than recommended upper limits (3 units per day for men and 2 units per day for women).

Pharmacological treatment

While there are very many drugs that can be used to lower blood pressure, four main classes of drugs will reduce blood pressure to target levels in the majority of patients:

- ACE inhibitors (and angiotensin receptor II blockers)
- Beta-blockers
- Calcium channel blockers
- Thiazide diuretics.

There are other classes of anti-hypertensive agent but their use is relatively rare:

- Vasodilator anti-hypertensives, including hydralazine and minoxidil
- Centrally acting anti-hypertensives, including clonidine and methyldopa
- Alpha-adrenoreceptors drugs such as doxazosin, indoramin and prazosin.

The most recent edition of the BHS guidelines recommend starting treatment with either an ACE, ARB or a beta-blocker for young (<55 years of age) and non-black patients. For others they recommend starting treatment with either a calcium channel blocker or a thiazide diuretic. If blood pressure is not controlled on this treatment, as may be the case in a majority of patients, a stepwise increase in treatment is recommended as outlined in Fig. 5.2, known as the 'AB-CD algorithm'.

The choice of antihypertensive needs also to take into account any other disease suffered by the patient, which is the case for a great many patients with hypertension. Guidelines on this issue are usually provided in terms of what drugs are strongly indicated (compelling indications), what drugs are potentially useful (possible indications), which drugs are not advised (cautions) and drugs that ought not be used (compelling contraindications). These are summarised in Table 5.2.

In addition to the treatment of their hypertension, patients may benefit from treatment with other agents that reduce the risk of cardiovascular events, particularly aspirin and statins.

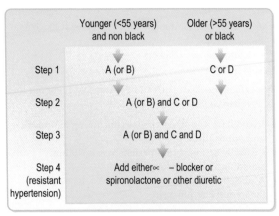

Key:A = ACE inhibitor or angiotensin II receptor blocker, B = beta-blocker, C = calcium channel blocker and D = thiazide or thiazide like diuretic

Fig. 5.2 **The AB-CD algorithm for treatment of hypertension**

Table 5.2
Pharmacological treatments for hypertension

Class of drug	Compelling indications	Possible indications	Caution	Compelling contraindications
α-blockers	Benign prostatic hypertrophy Heart failure Left ventricular dysfunction Type 1 diabetic nephropathy Secondary prevention of IHD and stroke		Postural hypotension Renal impairment Peripheral vascular disease	Urinary incontinence Pregnancy Reno-vascular disease
ACE inhibitors		Chronic renal disease Type II diabetic nephropathy Proteinuric renal disease		
Angiotensin II receptor blockers	ACE inhibitor intolerance Type 2 diabetic nephropathy Hypertension with LVH Heart failure post-MI in patients intolerant of ACE inhibitor	LVF post-MI Intolerance of other anti-hypertensives Proteinuric disease Chronic renal failure Heart failure	Renal impairment Peripheral vascular disease	Pregnancy Reno-vascular disease

Table 5.2 Continued.

Class of drug	Compelling indications	Possible indications	Caution	Compelling contraindications
β-blockers	Myocardial infarction Angina	Heart failure	Heart failure Peripheral vascular disease Diabetes (except with IHD)	Asthma or COPD Heart block
Calcium channel blockers (dihydropyridine)	Elderly Isolated systolic hypertension	Angina		
Calcium channel blockers (other)	Angina	Elderly	Combination with β-blockers	Heart block, heart failure
Thiazide diuretics	Elderly Isolated systolic hypertension Heart failure Secondary stroke prevention			Gout

174

Complications

The cardiovascular, renal and ophthalmic complications of hypertension are noted above under clinical features.

Monitoring

The frequency of follow-up of patients with high blood pressure will depend on the severity and variability of blood pressure, the complexity of the treatment regimen, and the need to give or reinforce lifestyle advice. It is suggested that patients whose blood pressure is reasonably stable be reviewed every 6 months. Sitting blood pressure and weight should be recorded at each visit. For older patients and patients with diabetes the blood pressure should be measured both sitting and standing to check for postural hypotension. Urine should be checked for protein annually. Enquiry into the possible development of adverse effects of

---

Box 5.9 Process measures of performance in hypertension management

- What proportion of the practice population over 50 have had blood pressure measured in the past 1, 3 and 5 years?
- What proportion of the population with hypertension who smoke and/or drink have been offered appropriate lifestyle advice?
- What proportion of patients with hypertension are on one or more appropriate medication(s)?
- What proportion of patients with hypertension have been reviewed in the previous 6 and 12 months?
- What proportion of patients on treatment for hypertension have a recent reading within their target range?
- Proportion of patients for whom aspirin and/or statins are receiving these medicines?
- Proportion of patients who have had urinalysis for protein within the last year?
- Proportions of patients on diuretics, ACEIs or ARBs who have had urea, electrolytes or creatinine levels checked within the last year?

medicines should be made and bloods should be taken to monitor urea, electrolytes and creatinine levels. Lifestyle factors such as diet, physical activity levels, tobacco and alcohol consumption should also be reviewed. Patient compliance with their medicines should also be checked.

What the patient should know

Patients need to know that hypertension is just one risk factor for cardiovascular disease. They need to be encouraged to take all necessary steps to reduce their cardiovascular risk, including adhering to whatever lifestyle advice is given and whatever pharmacological treatment is offered. Patients should be told what their blood pressure readings are and what their target level is. However, it may not be advisable for patients to obtain their own blood pressure monitor, as many monitors sold to patients do not meet BHS criteria for reliability of reading. Also, patients with their own monitors may become obsessive about measuring their blood pressure, to little benefit.

Primary care team

An appropriately trained practice nurse can do a good deal of the monitoring and follow-up of patients with

Box 5.10   New GP (UK) contract requirements/
indicators for hypertension

- BP 1. The practice can produce a register of patients with established hypertension
- BP 2. The percentage of patients with hypertension whose notes record smoking status at least once
- BP 3. The percentage of patients with hypertension who smoke, whose notes contain a record that smoking cessation advice has been offered at least once
- BP 4. The percentage of patients with hypertension in which there is a record of the blood pressure in the past 9 months
- BP 5. The percentage of patients with hypertension in whom the last blood pressure (measured in last 9 months) is 150/90 or less

hypertension. Patients who have difficulties with maintaining an appropriate diet may benefit from seeing a dietician.

Performance review

To review the care of hypertension a practice should review its record for evidence of the process and outcome measures listed in Box 5.9. The contract requirements are listed in Box 5.10.

Asthma

Essential background

Asthma is a respiratory condition associated with inflammation and reversible limitation of airflow. It is very common, occurring in 30% of children and 8% of adults in the UK.

Diagnosis/definition

Asthma has been defined as a difference of at least 15% between peak flow readings taken on two different occasions.

Clinical features

The quintessential clinical feature of asthma is wheeze, but cough and a sensation of tightness in the chest or difficulty in breathing are also common features. Symptoms are typically worse at night and may be precipitated or exacerbated by cold, exercise and a variety of allergens such as animal dander, house-dust mite, and pollen. Physical examination is often normal at the time of presentation to a general practitioner but signs of respiratory distress, particularly indrawing of the subcostal area, use of accessory muscles of respiration and an elevated respiratory rate, may occur – particularly during acute attacks.

Pulse rate may also be elevated, though this may be contributed to by overuse of bronchodilators. Pallor or cyanosis, inability to talk and 'silent chest' are all very ominous features – indicating the need for immediate administration of oxygen and referral to hospital. In milder exacerbations or sometimes on presentation rhonchi may be present. Peak flow readings may be below those expected for the patient's age, height and gender and may be normal when seen in the clinic but drop at other times. Therefore, it is useful to give the patient a peak flow meter to take serial readings at different times of the day and night.

A reversibility test in which peak flow is measured before and after a dose of a bronchodilator may also be useful in showing up reversible airways obstruction. An exercise provocation test in which peak flow is measured before and after vigorous exercise may also be diagnostically useful.

Management

Detailed guidelines on the management of asthma are published by the British Thoracic Society and have been adopted by the Scottish Inter-collegiate Guidelines Network (www. sign.ac.uk). The key points only are summarised here.

Non-pharmacological management

Once asthma has developed the patient will usually require pharmacological treatment. However, there are some measures that may reduce the risk of developing asthma or may reduce the frequency and severity of attacks. These principally relate to avoidance of allergens and pollutants. Common allergens that may provoke asthma are pollen, house-dust mite and animal danders – minimisation of these in the environment is usually helpful.

Of various pollutants postulated to provoke asthma only cigarette smoking and sulphur dioxide (typically from burning of coal) occur commonly – avoidance of exposure to these has been shown to benefit patients with asthma. Thus patients with asthma who smoke must be urged and assisted to quit, while parents of children with asthma should be urged to either quit – or at least avoid smoking in the environment shared with their asthmatic children.

Breast feeding has been shown to be associated with a reduced risk of the development of wheeze in infants. Certain drugs may provoke or exacerbate asthma, particularly beta-blockers and non-steroidal anti-inflammatories, and these must be avoided in patients with asthma.

Pharmacological management

The essence of the BTS guidelines is a step-wise approach to management with treatment stepped up to the next level of pharmacotherapy if the symptoms are not controlled with the treatment given.

Step 1 – Mild intermittent asthma All patients with symptoms of asthma benefit from an inhaled bronchodilator. Inhaled bronchodilators are preferable to alternative formulations such as syrup. Patients on inhaled bronchodilators need to have their consumption of these monitored. If use exceeds two canisters per month or 10–12 puffs per day they need to be reviewed and considered for inhaled steroid treatment.

Step 2 – Regular preventer therapy Patients not controlled on intermittent bronchodilator treatment, which may be the majority of patients, should be started on an inhaled corticosteroid. These should be administered twice daily, although once-daily treatment at the same total dose may be considered once control has been achieved. Children on regular inhaled steroids should have their height monitored.

Step 3 – Add-on therapy If asthma is not controlled on low-dose inhaled steroids – and after checking compliance, inhaler technique and eliminating exposure to possible allergens or pollutants – add-on therapy should be considered. The first add-on treatment to be considered should be a long-acting beta-agonist such as salmeterol. If control is not achieved, inhaled steroid doses should be increased to a maximum of 800 µg/day of beclometasone (or equivalent doses of alternative inhaled steroids) in adults and 400 µg/day in children from the age of 5 years. Where there is no response to a long-acting beta-agonist an alternative add-on treatment such as a leukotriene receptor antagonist or a theophylline may be tried at this stage. If control is still not achieved this is deemed persistent poor control and treatment progresses to step 4.

> **Step 4 – Persistent poor control** Several options for the next step exist – as yet there is no clear evidence to indicate which is best. One option is to increase inhaled steroids to a maximum of 2000µg/day of beclometasone or equivalent in adults and 800µg/day in children over 5 years. Alternatively, start the patient on a leukotriene receptor antagonist or on a theophylline. For patients not already on an inhaled long-acting beta-agonist (which would only arise when this had been tried at step 3 and been ineffective) an oral long-acting beta-agonist might be tried.

Step 5 – Continuous or frequent use of oral steroids Patients whose asthma is not controlled by the above measures will usually require oral steroids, although some may also be managed on combinations of the step 4 drugs. However, management beyond step 4 is usually considered beyond the scope of general practice.

Use of inhalers

Another important aspect of the management of asthma is the use of the various inhaler devices available. Most inhaled asthma treatments are best taken using a metered dose inhaler in combination with a spacer device such as a Volumatic. Patients need to be trained by a competent health professional in order to be able to use their inhaler effectively. Getting an effective dose from a metered dose inhaler without the aid of a spacer device is difficult for many people. Other devices may be preferred by some patients, especially where they may have to administer their inhaled medicine outside the home. Whatever device is chosen, a check should be made to see that the patient can use the device properly.

The treatment of acute asthma is touched on in Chapter 3 but further details are available as part of the BTS guidelines (www.brit-thoracic.org.uk). Patients with asthma should receive pneumococcal immunisation once and annual influenza immunisation.

Complications

The main complication of asthma is the occurrence of acute attacks. These may occur for a variety of reasons but common precipitants include respiratory tract infections (especially viral upper respiratory tract infections in children), exposure to allergens or pollutants, or non-adherence to prescribed treatment.

Treatments used in asthma management can also cause adverse effects, which might also be considered complications. Candida infection of the throat or mouth and dysphonia occur with inhaled corticosteroids, especially if a metered dose inhaler is used without a spacer. The risk of these complications can be reduced by rinsing out the mouth after dosing. Growth retardation in children on inhaled steroids is also a concern – although at normal doses this can usually be avoided and final height is usually unaffected. Other complications associated with higher doses of steroids include osteoporosis, cataracts and adrenal suppression.

Monitoring

Patients with asthma should be kept under regular review, although the frequency will depend on the stability of the condition. The review visit should examine the frequency and extent of symptoms suffered since the last review. Specific enquiry should be made about wheeze, cough and chest tightness. There should also be some specific enquiry about nocturnal symptoms as they, even in the absence of daytime symptoms, indicate incomplete control. Likewise, ask about exercise-induced symptoms. Although a respiratory system examination should be conducted, the key measure of control is the peak expiratory flow rate measured with a peak flow meter. Ideally, though, the patient should have a personal peak flow meter (these can be prescribed to patients in the UK on the NHS) and take readings at different times of day and night, particularly prior to a clinic review or if there is any deterioration in symptoms. These readings should be looked at during a review visit.

Another major issue in the review process is inhaler techniques. Patients should be asked to bring all their inhalers and spacers to clinic and should be directly observed taking a dose of inhaler in the clinic. Any errors of technique should be corrected – but without making the patient feel bad about having 'got it wrong'. Ask about how and when they take their medicines. Ascertain how well the patient understands the medication – in particular, understanding the different use of 'preventer' and 'reliever' medicines should be checked and the patient should be given guidance on how and when to increase and decrease the dose in relation to symptoms and possible provocations of asthma (such as exercise).

Primary healthcare team
- Practice nurse
- Pharmacist – education re nature and use of medications including checking and reinforcement of inhaler technique
- Specialist/liaison/outreach asthma/pulmonary care nurse(s).

The patient's role
- Needs to understand nature and provoking factors in asthma and, especially, of acute attacks
- Use inhalers as recommended
- Self-monitoring with own peak flow meter
- May need to adjust the doses of inhalers
- Adherence to lifestyle and other advice
- Self-help group – The Asthma Society.

Performance review (audit)
See Box 5.11 for the process and proxy measures of GP practice performance and Box 5.12 for the GP contract requirements.

Chronic obstructive pulmonary disease

Essential background information

As the name suggests, chronic obstructive pulmonary disease (COPD) is a condition associated with chronic

Box 5.11 Process and proxy measures of asthma management

Process measures

- Number of patients on the asthma register – compared to number receiving relevant drugs and reported demographic norms
- Length of time since last review
- Proportion of asthma patients who smoke and of those the proportion who have had smoking cessation advice or treatment
- Proportion who have had the following checked:
  - Peak flow rate
  - Inhaler technique
- Proportions on different rungs of stepwise management hierarchy
- Proportion of patients immunised against pneumococcus ever and against influenza within last year

Proxy outcome measures

- Proportion of patients who require oral steroid course(s)
- Proportion of patients nebulised for asthma
- Proportion of patients hospitalised with asthma
- How long hospitalised for – length of stay

obstruction of airways. It is a broad-ranging term, which has been coined to encompass both chronic bronchitis and emphysema – which are now recognised as arising through common pathological processes and having considerable overlap in many patients.

Definition/diagnosis

- Chronic bronchitis has been defined as comprising chronic lung disease associated with production of sputum for at least 3 months of the year over the past 2 years
- Emphysema is defined as dilatation and destruction of lung tissue distal to the terminal bronchioles. This is the pathological definition. Emphysema is associated clinically mainly with breathlessness.

Box 5.12   New GP (UK) contract requirements/ indicators for asthma

- ASTHMA 1. The practice can produce a register of patients with asthma, excluding patients with asthma who have been prescribed no asthma-related drugs in the last 12 months
- ASTHMA 2. The percentage of patients age eight and over diagnosed as having asthma where the diagnosis has been confirmed by spirometry or peak flow measurement
- ASTHMA 3. The percentage of patients with asthma between the ages of 14 and 19 in whom there is a record of smoking status in the previous 15 months
- ASTHMA 4. The percentage of patients age 20 and over with asthma whose notes record smoking status in the past 15 months, except those who have never smoked where smoking status should be recorded at least once
- ASTHMA 5. The percentage of patients with asthma who smoke, and whose notes contain a record that smoking cessation advice has been offered within last 15 months
- ASTHMA 6. The percentage of patients with asthma who have had an asthma review in the last 15 months
- ASTHMA 7. The percentage of patients age 16 years and over with asthma who have had influenza immunisation in the preceding 1 September to 31 March

Clinical features

The key features of COPD are cough productive of sputum (associated with chronic bronchitis) and dyspnoea (the major symptom of emphysema). Wheeze is another major feature in many cases. Where wheeze is a major presenting feature, especially in younger patients, a distinction must be drawn between the possibilities of COPD and asthma. In asthma the wheeze is typically reversible, e.g. with bronchodilators, whereas in COPD the wheeze is not generally reversible –although one cannot be completely dogmatic about this as there may be a degree of reversibility of the wheeze in COPD.

COPD is also characterised by episodes of recurrent respiratory infection, mainly manifesting with increasing cough, increased sputum production (with sputum often becoming appreciably more purulent), increased wheeze, increased dyspnoea and, possibly, raised temperature. Smoking is a major aetiological factor in most patients with COPD – if they are not current smokers they will often have been heavy smokers in the past. COPD can also be associated with occupational exposure to inhaled toxins or irritants.

In mild cases of COPD there may be few signs but with progression of the disease audible rhonchi on chest auscultation become a more consistent feature. In severe COPD or during acute exacerbations there may be obvious respiratory distress with elevated respiratory rate and use of accessory muscles of respiration. In patients with respiratory failure (see Complications) there may be symptoms or signs of hypoxia (tachypnoea, confusion, etc.) or of hypercapnia (cyanosis, etc.). FEV_1 (forced expiratory volume in 1 second) is a key measurement in COPD and is used to classify the degree of severity of the disease as follows:

- mild COPD is defined as FEV_1 <80% of predicted
- moderate COPD is defined as FEV_1 <60% of predicted
- severe COPD is defined as FEV_1 <40% of predicted.

Management

Getting the patient to stop smoking is essential. While it will not reverse the loss of lung function it will slow the rate of deterioration in FEV_1 to a rate equivalent to that in non-smokers. Drug therapy likewise cannot stop the deterioration of lung function but is primarily aimed at reducing symptoms and the treatment of exacerbations. Treatment is guided by the severity of disease.

Mild disease without symptoms does not require drug therapy. Inhaled antimuscarinics or beta-agonists are used, according to clinical response, to relieve wheeze or dyspnoea. A trial of inhaled corticosteroids may be used to determine whether or not there is a steroid-responsive element to symptoms. For moderate disease the same treatments are used, though antimuscarinics and beta-agonists may also be used in combination, especially if there is a clinically useful response. Corticosteroids are also used if there is a useful response.

In severe disease long-acting beta-agonists will also be used and bronchodilator therapy is used on a more regular continuous basis. Corticosteroids usage is, again, determined by clinical response. Theophyllines are also tried in severe disease and continued if found useful.

Regular exercise is useful for patients with COPD and has been shown to increase exercise tolerance and improve quality of life. Obesity, if present, compounds the dyspnoea of COPD – obese patients should be offered assistance in weight reduction. Various forms of forced expiration and coughing exercises are also worthwhile in some cases. They will usually be initiated by a physiotherapist but, with instruction, may be continued by the patient at home.

Mucolytic agents may be useful in patients with frequent exacerbations but are not generally recommended for long-term use. Home oxygen therapy is used in advanced disease and, while it may prolong life, it has little or no benefit in relief of symptoms. Decisions about initiation of home oxygen are generally made in consultation with a specialist respiratory physician.

Acute infective exacerbations – indicated by increased dyspnoea, increased sputum production or purulent sputum – are generally treated with antibiotics. Appropriate antibiotics should be determined by local resistance patterns but local guidelines will usually include amoxicillin and a tetracycline. Oxygen therapy may also be beneficial, especially if arterial oxygen levels or pulse oximetry indicate hypoxia. However, care must be taken with dosage to avoid the risk of diminishing respiratory drive. Nebulised bronchodilators may also be beneficial. Short courses of oral corticosteroids (prednisolone 30–40 mg for 7–14 days) are also often used, especially if there has been previous evidence of symptoms being responsive to steroids.

Patients with COPD should also be vaccinated annually against influenza. They should also be immunised against pneumococcal disease. A non-type-specific *Haemophilus influenza* vaccine has also been tried in COPD but is not yet generally recommended.

Complications

The commonest complication of COPD is acute infective exacerbation (see above). Long-standing COPD can also lead to cor pulmonale (right ventricular failure).

Monitoring

FEV_1 is an important indicator of disease progression in patients with COPD and should be checked regularly. In addition, the pattern of symptoms should be enquired after at regular review, though patients should also know what symptoms indicate possible exacerbation (see above) and be encouraged to report when any such symptoms develop. The amount and colour of sputum production should be asked about at each review. While, ideally, arterial oxygen saturation would indicate the development of hypoxia this is not practical in general practice. A useful proxy measure of chronic hypoxia is the presence of polycythaemia on full blood count – its appearance may prompt specialist evaluation.

Naturally, if patients have not ceased smoking the amount they are smoking should be kept under review and continuing efforts made to encourage cessation. Patients' weight and exercise capacity should also be monitored and weight reduction and regular exercise encouraged where appropriate.

What the patient should know

Patients should realise that COPD is a chronic condition associated with irreversible lung damage. They should understand the likely role of smoking in the development of the condition (where this is the case) and should understand how important it is to quit smoking and remain abstinent. Patients should also understand the nature and likely precipitants of acute exacerbations and take steps to reduce the likelihood of exacerbations including regular exercise, avoiding smoky or polluted atmospheres, avoiding exposure to cold and damp conditions and appropriate use of any medicines prescribed. They should also know the symptoms that indicate the development of exacerbations and to seek medical attention when such symptoms occur. As the condition progresses they will need to understand the need for further therapies and, perhaps ultimately, the role of domiciliary oxygen.

Primary healthcare team
- GP
- Practice nurse
- Some specialist chest units may have a community-based pulmonary specialist nurse practitioner who, ideally, should work in close conjunction with the primary healthcare team.

Performance review
- Symptom inquiry at each visit
- Smoking status and whether smoking cessation advice/treatment has been offered
- FEV_1 readings at least annually
- Weight
- Exercise
- Haematocrit (for polycythaemia)
- Inhaler technique and symptom response to inhaler(s)
- Proportion of patients who have received pneumococcal immunisation ever and influenza immunisation within the last year.

See Box 5.13 for the contract requirements for management of COPD.

Osteoarthritis

Essential background information

Osteoarthritis is the commonest arthropathy in developed countries. It is associated with degenerative changes affecting weight-bearing joints particularly and it increases in prevalence with increasing age – although genetic, occupational and lifestyle factors affect prevalence too. The precise cause of osteoarthritis is unknown but trauma and

Box 5.13 New GP (UK) contract requirements/
indicators for COPD

- COPD 1. The practice can produce a register of patients
  with COPD
- COPD 2. The percentage of patients where diagnosis has
  been confirmed by spirometry including reversibility testing
  for newly diagnosed patients
- COPD 3. The percentage of all patients with COPD where
  diagnosis has been confirmed by spirometry including
  reversibility testing
- COPD 4. The percentage of patients with COPD in whom
  there is a record of smoking status in the previous 15
  months
- COPD 5. The percentage of patients with COPD who
  smoke, whose notes contain a record that smoking
  cessation advice has been offered in the past 15 months
- COPD 6. The percentage of patients with COPD with a
  record of FEV_1 in the previous 27 months
- COPD 7. The percentage of patients with COPD receiving
  inhaled treatment in whom there is a record that inhaler
  technique has been checked in the preceding 2 years
- COPD 8. The percentage of patients with COPD who have
  had influenza immunisation in the preceding 1 September
  to 31 March

189

mechanical damage are known to be significant factors in
its development and obesity is an important contributory
factor. In some cases there may be evidence of inflammation
in affected joints but this is not a universal feature.

Clinical features

The cardinal feature of osteoarthritis is pain in affected
joints. The joints most often affected are the hips and knees
but the joints of the hands are also often affected. It is also
quite common in the spine (both lumbar and cervical).
The pain is typically worse in the evenings and aggravated
by use of the affected joint(s). Stiffness occurs after a
period of rest but is short-lived (lasting 15–30 minutes),
unlike that associated with inflammatory arthritides such

as rheumatoid arthritis (see below). The disease is associated with progressive limitation of joint function and impairment of mobility.

Affected joints may be swollen and tender but are not usually red or hot, except in acute exacerbations. Acute exacerbations of osteoarthritis of the knee may be associated with patellar effusions or with Baker's cysts. Swellings may become permanent if they are due to bony overgrowth. In the hands swellings of the distal interphalangeal joints are known as 'Heberden's nodes', whereas swellings in the proximal interphalangeal joints are called 'Bouchard's nodes'.

X-ray changes associated with joint degeneration are the most pathognomonic feature of osteoarthritis but there is a poor correlation between X-ray changes and clinical severity. Changes include narrowing of joint spaces, periarticular sclerosis, bony cysts and osteophytes.

Management

The principal issues in the management of osteoarthritis are the relief of pain and the maintenance of mobility. Simple analgesics such as paracetamol and paracetamol in combination with various opiate derivatives are the mainstay of pharmacological treatment. Although NSAIDs are widely used in general practice they probably help mainly as analgesics rather than through any anti-inflammatory action – the role of inflammation in the disease process of osteoarthritis is disputed. There is no evidence of any long-term benefit from NSAID treatment and they are potentially dangerous in elderly patients (who make up the bulk of OA sufferers) because of their gastrointestinal side effects.

Glucosamine (Dona) is proposed as a disease modifying drug which, taken long-term, is said to limit progression of joint degeneration. Evidence supporting its use in this indication is, as yet, limited. It has been shown to be equal in efficacy to NSAIDs in terms of providing symptom relief. During exacerbations with severe pain stronger analgesics such as tramadol may be required. Intra-articular injections with corticosteroids can also be helpful in severe exacerbations affecting single accessible joints such as the knee.

Weight loss in obese patients is an important part of management and a dietician, if available, may be able to help with this. Physiotherapists also have a lot to offer OA patients both in terms of symptom relief with various forms of heat therapy and in improving mobility through muscle-strengthening exercises. Physiotherapists and occupational therapists can also assist patients in obtaining various mobility aids and in rehabilitation after surgery. Joint replacement surgery has proven particularly successful in the management of OA of the hip. Other forms of joint replacement are available with increasingly good results. Further surgical options include arthrodeses and osteotomies.

Monitoring

Patients with OA should be reviewed regularly to check they are receiving adequate analgesia but also to monitor mobility. Overweight patients will need to have their weight monitored. There are specific questionnaires that can be used to quantify patients' level of functioning (e.g. Barthel's index) but a general review of how the patient goes about their activities of daily living will give a good idea of how the disease is progressing and how well the patient is coping with any resultant disability. Various tests of joint and muscle strength can also be used to monitor disease progression.

What the patient should know

Patients need to know that they have a relatively benign form of arthritis that, while painful, is not generally life limiting. They also need to know that keeping up reasonable levels of activity is important as avoiding activity can contribute to increasing stiffness and muscle wasting – leading to a greater degree of immobility than would otherwise occur. Patients should also know about the effect of body mass on OA and be strongly encouraged to achieve and maintain ideal body weight for their height. They should also know about the possibility of joint replacement surgery – but this option should be reserved for when their degree of pain or disability merits the risks and discomforts of surgery.

Performance review

In performance review of the care of patients with OA the main issues are to check that patients are being encouraged to maintain activity levels and are receiving adequate analgesia. It should also be noted that patients have received adequate information about their disease and have had appropriate access to other primary care team members such as occupational therapy and physiotherapy.

Rheumatoid arthritis

Essential background information

Rheumatoid arthritis is the commonest of a group of conditions associated with abnormalities of the immune system and associated inflammation of connective tissues. Although most closely associated with an inflammatory arthritis, rheumatoid arthritis is a systemic disease with manifestations in many body systems. In order to stress this it is sometimes referred to as 'rheumatic' or 'rheumatoid' disease. Although the exact cause is unknown there are clearly genetic factors as it is associated strongly with having a positive family history and with the presence of certain genetically determined histocompatibility antigens (HLA-DR4 and HLA-D4).

Clinical features

Rheumatoid arthritis is characterised by joint pain, swelling and stiffness – particularly of the hands and feet – usually in a symmetrical pattern. Stiffness is usually most pronounced in the morning and usually wanes as the day goes on. The onset of the disease may be insidious or, occasionally, may present with an acute polyarthropathy associated with pyrexia and constitutional upset.

192

Inflamed joints may be red, hot and swollen during early attacks but over time characteristic deformities develop, including boutonniere and swan neck deformities of fingers, ulnar deviation of the fingers or hand, subluxations of affected joints, and muscle wasting of the small muscles of the hand. Corresponding deformities of the toes and feet may also occur. Periarticular features may also develop such as rheumatoid nodules of the extensor surfaces of elbows, at pressure points and along ligaments. Tenosynovitis and bursitis are other common manifestations.

Rheumatoid arthritis is a systemic disease – in addition to joint manifestations there are a large number of possible systemic manifestations that can occur (see Complications below). Laboratory testing for rheumatoid factors will be positive in 70% of cases (strongly so in most cases) and in 30% of cases anti-nuclear antibodies will also be present. X-rays are not strictly necessary in the making of the diagnosis but will typically show joint narrowing, erosion of joint margins, osteoporosis/osteopenia and lytic lesions or cysts in the bones. Full blood count may disclose a normochromic, normocytic anaemia while the ESR will usually be raised. Indeed, the ESR is a potentially useful gauge of the degree of inflammation, as is C reactive protein.

Management

Drugs used in the treatment of rheumatoid arthritis are divided into those that primarily relieve symptoms and those that are thought to alter the disease process itself – referred to as disease modifying agents (DMARDs). Commonly used symptom relievers include paracetamol with or without opiate agents; NSAIDs are also very widely used. DMARDs include corticosteroids, methotrexate, intra-articular or intramuscular gold injections, penicillamine and azathioprine. More recently developed drugs act to block the actions of tumour necrosis factor and include etanercept and infliximab (TNF alpha blockers). Many of these are associated with bone marrow toxicity and so full blood count needs regularly reviewed. Others are associated with either renal or hepatic damage – kidney and liver function also need to be kept under review.

Surgical treatment of joints to either prevent further progression or to try and reconstruct the joint is possible but decisions to operate must be weighed very carefully as surgery is not always successful in patients with this condition.

Complications

Pulmonary involvement may lead to effusions and pulmonary fibrosis, as well as rheumatoid nodules visible on chest X-ray. Vasculitis can result in nail-fold infarcts, leg ulcers and small areas of gangrene. Ocular complications include Sjögren's syndrome, uveitis and scleritis. Renal manifestations may be associated with amyloidosis. Neurological manifestations include carpal tunnel syndrome and other nerve entrapment syndromes including cord compression. Haematological manifestations are myriad but include anaemia and thrombocytosis. In juvenile arthritis hypersplenism and pancytopenia may occur in a condition called Felty's syndrome. Pericardial effusion and systemic features such as fever, fatigue and weight loss may also occur.

Monitoring

Disease progression should be monitored. The can be done by inquiry about symptoms but asking how the patient manages with activities of daily living can also give important indications of the incapacity caused by the disease – and hence severity. More formal test of grip strength and muscle power may also be useful to see if particular joints are getting better or worse with treatment. ESR and C reactive protein can also indicate the level of inflammation present at any time, which may guide anti-inflammatory treatment such as corticosteroids.

Other tests such as full blood count, renal and liver function tests are required to check for development of some of the more serious adverse effects of DMARDs. It is not practical to check for all possible systemic manifestations or complications at each visit but the patient should be encouraged to develop a low threshold to consult with other seemingly unrelated symptoms. Also, the doctor needs to have a high index of suspicion for these other manifestations of the disease process.

What the patient should know

The patient should know the nature of the condition, i.e. that it is a serious, usually progressive disease affecting joints primarily but with the possibility of various systemic manifestations. However, the patient should not be given an unduly gloomy prognosis. With modern treatments disease progression can be substantially impeded and the disease itself is very variable with remissions (sometimes lasting years) being common. Furthermore, the disease does tend to 'burn out' over time such that, while there may be varying degrees of joint deformity, pain will subside and the degree of residual function can be quite good. The patient also needs to know about the treatment and its major adverse reactions – if there are any such reactions the patient should stop taking the medicine (except steroids) and report to the doctor.

195

Primary healthcare team
- Physiotherapist – heat treatments, muscle strengthening exercises
- Occupational therapist – aids to living, adaptation of the patient's environment
- Social worker – guidance and assistance in obtaining appropriate benefits and grants.

Performance review
- Symptom status
- Adherence with medication and other treatments
- Proportions of patients on various medications
- Proportions of patients who have had the required blood tests at appropriate times.

Osteoporosis

Essential background information

Osteoporosis is a reduction in bone density associated with increased risk of fractures. Like hypertension it is, strictly speaking, not a disease per se, but rather a risk factor for a disease – the disease being pathological fracture.

Clinical features

Osteoporosis may be asymptomatic but some patients with osteoporosis may have pain in bones that are not fractured. Osteoporosis is associated with crush fractures of the vertebrae, which can result in dorsal kyphosis and exaggerated cervical lordosis (dowager's hump). Other commonly associated fractures are fractures of the neck of the femur and Colles' fractures of the wrist, but virtually any osteoporotic bone can fracture. Osteoporosis becomes more prevalent with increasing age and, in women, becomes particularly prevalent post-menopause. It also tends to run in families. Osteoporosis is diagnosed by means of bone densitometry using dual energy X-ray absorptiometry (DEXA) scanning. It is also often diagnosed retrospectively on X-ray once a fracture or fractures have occurred.

Management

The principal aim of management is to prevent fractures. Exercise and a diet rich in calcium are helpful, as is avoidance of smoking and excess alcohol consumption. Calcium supplements, however, usually in combination with vitamin D, are necessary to provide sufficient calcium to try and counteract the loss in bone density with age. These measures are all advisable in older patients – especially women – regardless of whether or not they have proven osteoporosis. Once osteoporosis is definitively established on DEXA scan using WHO criteria, further measures are usually required, which will include treatment with bisphosphonates, vitamin D, calcium supplements and possibly calcitonin. In postmenopausal women hormone replacement therapy may be recommended, or alternatively treatment with a SERM (selective oestrogen receptor modulator e.g. raloxifene) or a gonadomimetic (e.g. tibolone).

Complications

The main complications of osteoporosis are, obviously, fractures. Fractured neck of the femur is a particularly devastating complication because in elderly patients it is associated with quite a high level of morbidity and, indeed, mortality.

Monitoring

Patients with osteoporosis need regular (usually annual) DEXA scanning to monitor bone density. In addition, adherence to diet and exercise advice and to any prescribed medicines should be checked.

What the patient should know

Patients with osteoporosis need to understand that their condition is a risk factor for fractures in the future. They also need to understand that diet, exercise, and calcium supplementation are important elements of treatment in addition to prescribed medicines. Ideally, patients should understand that each medicine they take is designed to contribute to reducing their overall risk of fracture. Patients on bisphosphonates need to understand how to take these medicines to avoid oesophageal problems.

Performance review

The practice should know how many patients have had DEXA scans and what proportion of these have a diagnosis of osteoporosis. Furthermore, there should be a review of all patients with relevant fractures to ensure they have all been DEXA scanned. All patients with a diagnosis of osteoporosis should be reviewed to ensure that they are on the appropriate treatment and that they have scans at recommended intervals.

Psoriasis

Essential background information

Psoriasis is a chronic skin disease associated with overproduction of epidermal cells, inflammation and plaque formation. It varies greatly in extent from the presence of a few plaques to extensive disease affecting nearly all of the skin. It is known to have a familial incidence and is associated with certain specific HLA antigens. Its response to immunosuppressive therapy and the association with an arthropathy that resembles rheumatoid arthritis are suggestive of a possible immunological pathogenesis.

Clinical features

The characteristic lesion of psoriasis is a well-demarcated silvery scaly plaque, most typically occurring on the extensor surface of limbs. The scalp is also very often involved with scaly lesions and shedding of skin flakes that can be mistaken for dandruff. Characteristic nail changes may also be present with pitting and onycholysis. An arthropathy that resembles rheumatoid arthritis may occur – sometimes its development precedes the skin lesions. Guttate psoriasis is a less common form of the disease in which vesicular lesions occur. Pustular psoriasis is another rare form in which pustules are a prominent feature. Erythrodermic psoriasis is a generalised form with very extensive involvement and near universal scaling – this is a very rare but potentially life threatening form.

Management

There are a number of modalities for the treatment of psoriasis – which is applied will depend on the extent and severity of the disease. For disease limited to well-defined plaques local treatments will usually be the mainstay of treatment. These range from simple emollients, to creams and lotions containing coal tar, to calcipotriol (an analogue of vitamin D3) and ultimately to topical dithranol. Topical corticosteroids are also widely used and are quite effective but the lesions tend to recur once steroids are stopped. Long-term use of potent topical steroids is associated with irreversible thinning of the skin. For more severe and/or extensive disease oral retinoic acid derivatives and immunosuppressive therapies such as ciclosporin or methotrexate are used. An alternative treatment for severe disease is PUVA treatment, which involves oral administration of psoralens and exposure to ultraviolet A light. PUVA treatment is usually undertaken in hospital under supervision of a dermatologist.

Complications

- Erythrodermic (exfoliative) psoriasis
- Psoriatic arthropathy.

Monitoring

Psoriasis patients should be monitored for response to whatever treatment has been offered. Psoriasis is a naturally relapsing and remitting condition and it is not always possible or desirable to keep increasing the treatment in a quest for perfect skin. However, the range of treatments should be explored with the patient, with the aim of achieving a degree of control of the disease that is satisfactory to the patient. Patients on corticosteroids need to be checked for signs of steroid overuse. Those on retinoic acid treatments and immunosuppressive therapies need regular blood tests to check on liver function and haematology.

What the patient should know

The patient should understand that psoriasis is a chronic relapsing remitting condition in which total cure is not possible but where a good deal of control is generally possible. An understanding of the benefits and limitations of whatever treatment they are on is essential. Those using dithranol need to know to be careful not to apply it to normal skin – where it is a severe irritant. Patients using calcipotriol need to be aware of the danger of hypercalcaemia if this treatment is overused; those using corticosteroids need to be aware of the dangers of long-term steroid use. Female patients on retinoic acid derivatives need to know that these are highly teratogenic – it is vital they do not become pregnant while on this treatment or for at least 2 years after treatment ceases. Patients on immunosuppressive therapy need to understand the risks and the need to comply with blood test monitoring.

Performance review

A review of psoriasis management in the practice should be able to determine the number of patients on treatment for psoriasis in the practice and the treatments they are on. For each treatment used there should be a check that the appropriate monitoring (see above) is taking place and that the patient has been appropriately informed about the treatment.

Gastro-oesophageal reflux disease (GORD)

Essential background information

Gastro-oesophageal reflux disease is a name given to a condition associated with reflux of stomach acid into the lower end of the oesophagus. While there are many potential causes, the commonest is a sliding hiatus hernia. It is associated with obesity and with various conditions in which there is excess production of gastric acid including an irregular eating pattern, a high fat diet, smoking, excess alcohol consumption, bending and stooping, tight clothing and certain drugs such as non-steroidal anti-inflammatories, tricyclic anti-depressants, antimuscarinics and nitrates.

Clinical features

The principal presenting feature is heartburn which can comprise either a retrosternal burning sensation (typically on bending or stooping or after meals) and/or a sensation of acid or water (waterbrash) coming up the oesophagus and/or into the back of the throat or the mouth. Symptoms are often relieved by eating, cold or milky drinks and by antacids; they may be exacerbated by bending, stooping or lying down. Less commonly it may present with cough or wheeze, possibly due to leakage of stomach contents into the trachea.

Rarely it may present with haematemesis, anaemia or dysphagia (in which cases there is usually an associated oesophageal stricture). Barium swallow may reveal a hiatus hernia and upper GI tract endoscopy may reveal oesophagitis. The condition is, however, best diagnosed on clinical features.

Management

The aims of management are to relieve symptoms, promote healing of the oesophagus and prevent recurrence. Symptoms may be relieved by antacids and H_2 antagonists but the most effective drug treatment will usually be a proton pump inhibitor. However, to promote healing and reduce the risk of recurrence it is necessary to tackle underlying lifestyle factors such as diet, smoking, alcohol consumption, weight etc. Symptom relief may also be provided by sleeping with the head raised and by avoidance of overfilling the stomach. Stopping smoking and avoiding alcohol will also promote healing and reduce recurrence rates. Rarely, surgery with fundoplication may be needed.

Complications

- Anaemia
- Oesophageal stricture
- Barrett's oesophagus – metaplasia of the lower end of the oesophagus
- Oesophageal cancer – possibly secondary to Barrett's.

Monitoring

Patients should be reviewed regularly to ensure their condition is responding to any treatment prescribed and to ensure compliance. If there are persistent symptoms, full blood count may reveal any anaemia that might develop. Body weight should be kept under review – overweight or obese patients should be reviewed to check on progress in reducing weight.

What the patient should know

A patient with GORD needs to understand that they have a chronic but generally controllable condition. They particularly need to understand the substantial role played by lifestyle factors (diet, eating patterns, smoking, alcohol consumption etc.) in the genesis and perpetuation of this condition and, therefore, the importance of modifying their lifestyle to minimise the impact of this condition. Adherence to medication will usually be driven by symptoms anyway but patients should be discouraged from reliance on medication as a solution to their problem in preference to lifestyle modification – medication offers only a temporary and imperfect solution. A patient-by-patient judgement needs to be made about how much to highlight potential long-term complications of the disease to try and encourage patients to modify lifestyle.

Performance review

Review of the care of patients with GORD should focus on control of symptoms being achieved and effectiveness of patient education (see 'What the patient should know' above). In addition, though, it is important to check that all patients with the diagnosis of GORD have been properly investigated, i.e. the possibility of *Helicobacter pylori* infection having been excluded and endoscopy or barium swallow having been undertaken as appropriate to their age, symptoms and local guidelines on investigation use. Use of proton pump inhibitors (PPIs) in the practice is a good guide to the management of this and related conditions – review of prescribing data is a useful audit tool. Prescribing review should try and identify instances where PPIs and NSAIDs are being co-prescribed and such instances reviewed to check this prescribing is appropriate.

Hyperthyroidism

Essential background information

Hyperthyroidism is the condition resulting from an over-production of thyroid hormone from thyroid disease. There are several pathophysiological entities that can give rise to hyperthyroidism but the commonest is Graves' disease or diffuse toxic goitre. Graves' disease is an autoimmune condition in which antibodies are created that bind to TSH receptors within the thyroid gland – stimulating thyroid hormone production. Other causes of hyperthyroidism include toxic nodular goitre, subacute thyroiditis, Hashimoto's thyroiditis, and amiodarone therapy.

Clinical features

Typical features of hyperthyroidism include heat intolerance, sweating, tiredness and lethargy, tremor, muscle weakness, feelings of nervousness or anxiety, excessive sweating, breathlessness and palpitations, diarrhoea and weight loss. An enlarged thyroid gland (goitre) or a thyroid mass are common, but not invariable, signs. Tachycardia and even atrial fibrillation may occur, as well as other features of a haemodynamic circulation (flow murmurs and the like). There may be proximal myopathy with associated reduction in muscle power in proximal muscle groups. There may be a sore or gritty feeling in the eyes, diplopia, lid lag, and lid retraction in any form of hyperthyroidism but in Graves' disease there are more pronounced features of exophthalmos. Pre-tibial myxoedema on the shin is another feature specific to Graves' disease. Hyperthyroidism is occasionally discovered as result of routine blood testing.

Management

There are three main forms of treatment of hyperthyroidism – anti-thyroid drugs, partial or total ablation of the thyroid gland with radioactive iodine, and surgery. The main anti-thyroid drugs are carbimazole and propylthiouracil. Both are prone to causing neutropenia but this usually develops in the first 8 weeks of treatment and so is closely monitored for over this time. Remission does not occur in all cases and relapse is common. Most patients go on to ablative therapy with radioactive iodine. Surgery is deployed nowadays as a treatment of last resort if there is poor response to other treatments – it is more strongly indicated where the patient has a large or unsightly goitre. Thyroid eye disease may need treatment with artificial tears, sunglasses, and, possibly, diuretics. Occasionally peri-orbital surgery or ocular radiotherapy is required to relieve symptoms and/or conserve sight. Monitoring of thyroid function is required during and after all forms of management.

Complications

- Exophthalmos
- Atrial fibrillation
- Goitre
- Hypothyroidism (due to overshoot in ablative therapies).

Monitoring

Thyroid function needs to be kept under regular review to ensure that the patient is not drifting into hypothyroidism – a common occurrence. Pulse should also be taken to gauge thyroid function and to exclude atrial fibrillation. The patient should also be reviewed with regard to level of adherence to their treatment.

What the patient should know

Patients should know they have an 'overactive' thyroid. They should also know that it can be controlled by medication, providing it is taken properly as prescribed.

Performance review

- Thyroid function tests including TSH
- Compliance with treatment.

Hypothyroidism

Essential background information

Hypothyroidism arises when there is a deficiency in the production of thyroid hormone. It is most often due to autoimmune thyroiditis but can be secondary to surgery or iodine treatment for hyperthyroidism, drugs such as amiodarone or lithium, viral thyroiditis or, rarely, pituitary disease. Historically, iodine deficiency was a common cause of hypothyroidism, especially in inland areas.

Clinical features

Typical features of hypothyroidism include cold intolerance, hoarseness, constipation, weight gain, dry skin, thinning of hair, facial puffiness, bradycardia, nerve entrapment syndromes such as carpal tunnel syndrome, and slow relaxing ankle reflexes. Iodine deficiency and Hashimoto's thyroiditis may be associated with a goitre but other forms of hypothyroidism may not be. Hypothyroidism may also present with a variety of psychiatric conditions including depression and psychosis ('myxoedema madness'). It can also be a cause of menorrhagia and infertility. Very often, though, it is picked up on blood tests in patients with vague complaints such as fatigue. Typically, it is associated with a high TSH level and low T4, although in deficiencies of thyroid binding globulin or pituitary disease it may present with low T4 with a normal TSH.

Management

Hypothyroidism is treated with thyroxine. Treatment is started with low doses of thyroxine, which are gradually built up until a normal T4 level is achieved and TSH is suppressed to normal levels. The biochemical improvement will usually precede clinical recovery – close monitoring of thyroid function tests during early treatment is required. Once stabilised, thyroid function still needs to be checked at regular (annual) intervals.

Complications

Untreated hypothyroidism is associated with increased risk of ischaemic heart disease. Severe hypothyroidism is associated with a rare but life threatening condition called myxoedema coma in which the patient, typically an elderly person, presents with coma and hypothermia in the presence of very low levels of thyroid hormone.

Monitoring

Once diagnosed with hypothyroidism thyroid function tests (i.e. T4 and TSH) need to be performed regularly – usually once per year. Clinical manifestations (see above) should also be checked for. In view of the association of hypothyroidism with lipid disorders, fasting blood lipids should also be monitored. Replacement therapy with thyroxine is the cornerstone of management – compliance with treatment should also be reviewed regularly.

What the patient should know

Patients should understand that they have a hormone deficiency syndrome – which is easily and fully correctable with replacement therapy. They must understand that replacement therapy is lifelong and that, in view of the lack of a close correlation between clinical symptoms and blood levels of thyroxine, they should only adjust the dosage of their medicine in consultation with their doctor.

Performance review

In reviewing the management of hypothyroidism in a practice it is important to check on the proportion of patients known to have hypothyroidism who are in receipt of regular prescriptions for thyroxine at appropriate intervals (depending on the repeat prescribing system in operation). It is also important to check the proportion of these patients who have had thyroid function checked within the last year – and the proportion of these whose thyroid function tests results are normal (see Box 5.14).

Box 5.14   New GP (UK) contract requirements/
indicators for hypothyroidism

- THYROID 1. The practice can produce a register of patients with hypothyroidism
- THYROID 2. The percentage of patients with hypothyroidism with thyroid function tests recorded in the previous 15 months

Epilepsy

Essential background information

Epilepsy is the condition of having a tendency to recurrent seizures. Seizures take a variety of forms of which the most common – grand mal – is associated with loss of consciousness and tonic–clonic movements of the body. Other forms of seizures are petit mal, in which there are short-lived lapses in consciousness and cessation of activity (which occur mainly in children); Jacksonian or partial seizures, in which the motor symptoms are often confined, at least initially, to part of the body such as a limb; and temporal lobe epilepsy, which is associated with hallucinations and other psychological symptoms.

Clinical features

Seizures are, obviously, the main clinical feature of epilepsy but initially it can be difficult to distinguish epilepsy from other forms of temporary unconsciousness such as simple fainting (vasovagal attacks). Given the serious consequences for the patient of a diagnosis of epilepsy, the diagnosis should, ideally, be made on the basis of a good eyewitness account of the seizure confirmed by EEG and/or neurological opinion. In grand mal epilepsy the tonic–clonic movements may be associated with urinary and/or faecal incontinence. During fits patients may damage themselves on objects if these are in the way of flailing limbs. Patients may also bite or swallow their tongue and efforts should be made to avoid such compromise to the airway of a patient in a fit. After a grand mal fit the patient may feel very drowsy or may go to sleep. In Jacksonian epilepsy there may be paralysis of the affected limb after a fit – Todd's paralysis. Hallucinations in temporal lobe epilepsy may be visual or olfactory.

It is important to remember that epilepsy is not a disease, per se, but may be a manifestation of some form of neurological damage. Therefore, it is also important to look for possible causes of epilepsy, which can include cerebrovascular disease, encephalitis, various toxins (including alcohol), and intracranial space-occupying lesions such as brain tumours and abscesses.

Management

The main anti-epileptic drugs and their key features are outlined in Table 5.3. Most patients with epilepsy will be successfully controlled with monotherapy but a minority of patients will require combination therapy with two anti-

Table 5.3
Main anti-epileptic drugs

Drug	Features
Phenytoin	Used in all forms of epilepsy. It has a very narrow therapeutic index and requires careful dose adjustment. Causes gum hyperplasia, hirsuitism, acne and coarse facies. Toxicity is associated with drowsiness, ataxia and nystagmus.
Carbamazepine	Drug of choice for simple and complex partial seizures and for tonic–clonic seizures with a focal discharge. Fewer side effects than phenytoin and a wider therapeutic index. Adverse effects include blurred vision, dizziness, nausea, headache and a rash. It is an enzyme inducer and interacts with a wide range of medicines, including other anti-epileptics.
Valproate	Used in generalised or partial seizures. Main side effects include nausea, weight gain (it stimulates appetite), hair loss with thin curly re-growth, ataxia, and tremor. It can cause liver damage, blood disorders and pancreatitis and patients on valproate require close monitoring of liver and marrow function before and after commencing treatment.
Ethosuximide	Used mainly in simple absence seizures (petit mal). Adverse effects include gastric disturbances, weight loss, drowsiness, headache and ataxia. Requires monitoring of liver, renal and marrow function.
Lamotrigine	Used for generalised and partial seizures. Main side effect is a rash. Initially developed as an adjunct treatment it is increasingly used as a sole treatment.

Table 5.3 *Continued.*

Drug	Features
Vigabatrin	Used mainly for partial seizures and in combination with other anti-epileptic drugs. Main side effect is occurrence of visual field defects – requires close monitoring of visual fields. Also causes behavioural side effects in some patients.
Gabapentin	Used mainly as an adjunct or add-on therapy for partial seizures. Also used in treatment of neuropathies. Main adverse effects include drowsiness, dizziness, ataxia, and fatigue.
Topiramate	Used as an adjunctive treatment for partial seizures and for generalised tonic–clonic seizures not controlled with other drugs. Adverse effects include abdominal pain, nausea, weight loss, mood disorders, behavioural disorders and visual disturbances.

epileptic drugs. The choice of therapy is guided by type of epilepsy, adverse effects of drugs and interactions between drugs. Choosing the correct drug or combination of drugs is a specialist area and, ideally, should be undertaken by a neurologist with a special interest in epilepsy.

The management of the patient with epilepsy is about much more than getting the right drug or drug combination to control fits. Having epilepsy is a stigmatising condition that has major implications in many aspects of patients' lives. It may affect capacity for employment and driving. The vehicle licensing authorities publish detailed guidelines on which patients with epilepsy may or may not drive. It may also restrict social lives as patients cannot drink alcohol and fits may be induced by lack of sleep.

Patients with epilepsy have an understandable concern over the potential for the condition to be hereditary and it has implications for reproduction, as many of the drugs are potentially teratogenic. Management of epilepsy in pregnancy is very challenging. As epilepsy is a condition associated with stigma it causes many psychological problems for patients and creates a range of difficulties for patients, particularly around whom to tell and not tell about their condition. Patients need a lot of psychosocial support in which the primary healthcare team can play a vital role.

Complications

Status epilepticus is a condition of continuous fitting that can occur in patients with epilepsy. It is a life-threatening emergency. Secure the patient's airway and treat with oxygen and intravenous or rectal diazepam or lorazepam.

Monitoring

All patients with epilepsy need regular monitoring, primarily to ensure they are remaining fit-free or at least that fits are being kept to a minimum by their drug regimen. If fits are occurring, compliance with drug therapy should be checked and a detailed history may be needed to determine if there are particular circumstances in which fits are occurring. Some patients may need regular blood tests to determine the blood level of their anti-epileptic but this is less necessary if fits are under control and there are no apparent adverse effects from the drugs. For many of the drugs, patients will also need regular monitoring of hepatic, renal and/or marrow function (see above).

Given the myriad psychological effects of epilepsy it is also important to monitor patients' mental health, to ensure that they are coping with their epilepsy and that it is not interfering with their lives to any greater extent than is unavoidable.

What the patient should know

Patients should understand the nature of epilepsy, i.e. that it is a long-term condition probably associated with some form of neurological damage but that it is usually controllable on medication – which they must continue to take until advised it is safe to stop. If there is an established cause of their epilepsy the patients should be informed of this too. Patients need to know whether or not they are permitted to drive and the licensing authorities' guidelines on this should be consulted. They should understand that epilepsy, if controlled, should not interfere unduly in the conduct of their lives but that they may be precluded from certain occupations (in which having a fit would constitute a grave danger to themselves or others) and may need to avoid certain activities including extreme or adventure sports and consumption of alcohol.

Women of child-bearing years need to know that while becoming pregnant is manageable they need to inform their doctors before embarking on a pregnancy and will need close attention to their medicines and other aspects of their illness during the pregnancy.

Performance review

The practice ought to keep a register of patients with epilepsy. In a performance review it should be determined which patients are on which drugs and if all patients are receiving the blood test monitoring appropriate to their drug(s). The proportion of known epilepsy sufferers who have been fit-free for over a year is a good outcome indicator, although it may not be entirely reflective of the success of the practice in managing epilepsy. The proportion of adult patients who have been informed of their status vis-a-vis capacity to drive should also be recorded (see Box 5.15).

Box 5.15   New GP (UK) contract requirements/indicators for epilepsy

- EPILEPSY 1. The practice can produce a register of patients receiving drug treatment for epilepsy
- EPILEPSY 2. The percentage of patients age 16 and over on drug treatment for epilepsy who have a record of seizure frequency in the previous 15 months
- EPILEPSY 3. The percentage of patients age 16 and over on drug treatment for epilepsy who have a record of medication review in the previous 15 months
- EPILEPSY 4. The percentage of patients age 16 and over on drug treatment for epilepsy who have been convulsion-free for last 12 months recorded in last 15 months

Further Reading

Ballinger A, Patchett S 2003 Saunders' pocket essentials of clinical medicine, 3rd edn. W B Saunders, Edinburgh

Cartwright S, Goodlee C 2003 Churchill's pocketbook of general practice, 2nd edn. Churchill Livingstone, Edinburgh

Department of Health 2003 Investing in general practice: the new general medical services contract. The Stationery Office, London

Khot A, Polmear A 2003 Practical general practice, 4th edn. Butterworth Heinemann, Edinburgh

Kumar P, Clark M 2002 Clinical medicine, 5th edn. W B Saunders, Edinburgh

Murtagh J 2003 General practice, 3rd edn. McGraw Hill, New York

6 Health promotion and disease prevention

The traditional role of the doctor has been to respond to health problems presented by people who are ill or believe themselves to be ill. However, it is increasingly recognised that doctors also have a valuable role in the prevention of disease and the promotion of health. As the understanding of the antecedent causes and causative factors underlying many common diseases advances, the scope for prevention increases. There are three types of disease prevention activity undertaken by general practitioners, as illustrated in Table 6.1.

Besides these specific preventive activities targeted at particular illnesses, health promotion is also about maintaining and promoting health in the broader World Health Organization (WHO) sense of health as complete physical, psychological and social wellbeing. Health promotion, therefore, includes disease prevention, health education, policies which promote healthy living and a host of other activities which all share the goal of maximising health in this positive and holistic sense. Health promotion involves very many people and agencies including, but not confined

Table 6.1
Types of prevention and general practice examples

Type of prevention	Nature of preventive activity	General practice example
Primary	Preventing disease before it happens	Immunisation
Secondary	Preventing asymptomatic disease progressing to symptomatic disease	Cervical cytology screening
Tertiary	Prevention of complications of established disease	Cardiac rehabilitation post myocardial infarction

to, those in the identifiable health services. Among doctors, GPs make a particularly valuable contribution because:

- GPs have an established relationship of trust with the patient, which makes them a credible and dependable source of advice.
- Patients see their GPs as having a general and legitimate interest in their health and so they are more accepting of the GP's role in advising and intervening regarding health issues that the patients might not have specifically raised.
- GPs have many opportunities for health promotion as, on average, about two-thirds of a practice population will visit their GP on at least one occasion over a 12-month period and over 90% will have visited over a 5-year period.

Health surveillance and screening

Screening is advocated for a wider and wider range of health problems – but not all screening programmes are equally worthwhile. Which of the various health-screening manoeuvres might or might not be worthwhile has been widely considered and criteria for determining which are worth

> **Box 6.1** Summary of Wilson's criteria for the establishment of a screening programme
>
> **Disease-related criteria**
> - Disease is a significant public health problem
> - The natural history of the disease is well understood
> - There is an identifiable pre-clinical stage
>
> **Test-related criteria**
> - There is a suitable screening test with good specificity and sensitivity
> - The screening test must be acceptable
> - There is a suitable and acceptable diagnostic test
>
> **Treatment-related criteria**
> - There is a treatment which instituted early reduces risk of progression to more serious disease
>
> **Economic criteria**
> - The whole programme of screening tests, diagnostic tests and treatment should be deemed economically viable
> - The appropriate treatment must be available
> - Appropriate treatment facilities must be available
> - There is a protocol on who to treat
>
> **Other criteria**
> - The benefits must outweigh the cost on a population basis
> - There is a continuing political commitment to the programme

doing were first proposed by Wilson (see Further Reading) and subsequently adopted by the WHO (Box 6.1).

Disease criteria

The disease for which a screening procedure is proposed should pose a reasonably serious risk to health – ischaemic heart disease would be worthwhile while ingrowing toenails would not be. The disease needs to be reasonably common – although if it is serious enough and the test is reasonably cheap a lot of people may be screened even for a relatively rare disease. Thus, while it might be technically possible to screen for acromegaly it would be difficult to justify screening because it is so rare and the test for it (growth hormone level) is expensive. However, phenylketonuria is a relatively rare disease and yet young babies are routinely screened for this condition because the screening test (the Guthrie heel prick test) is quite cheap, the disease is simply and cheaply treated (with a special diet) and the consequences of untreated disease are quite devastating.

The disease must have an early or latent phase during which it can be picked up by the screening test. An example of a disease with an early or latent phase is cervical cancer, which is preceded by pre-invasive carcinoma-in-situ that can be detected by cervical cytological testing (the Pap smear). The disease should have a reasonably well-understood natural history. Cervical cytology does not do so well on this criteria as we are unsure how often pre-invasive disease proceeds to become invasive, nor do we know the usual time-scale for this development to occur.

Test criteria

Tests may be characterised by their sensitivity and specificity for a particular disease. A test that is very *sensitive* will nearly always be positive when the disease is present (i.e. few false-negatives) but may also sometimes be positive even in the absence of disease (i.e. a high false-positive rate). By contrast, a highly *specific* test has a low probability of being positive if the disease is absent (few false-positives) but it may be negative in some cases where the disease is present (i.e. a high false-negative rate) (Table 6.2).

Rarely do tests have both high sensitivity and specificity and often one is traded off against the other. However, to be used in screening asymptomatic people, a screening test or procedure must have a reasonably high sensitivity and

216

Table 6.2
Features typical of sensitive and specific tests

Type of test	False-negative rate	False-positive rate
Sensitive tests	low	high
Specific tests	high	low

specificity for the disease. The test must also be acceptable to people without symptoms. For instance, it has been proposed that digital rectal examination could be used to screen for possible prostate cancer in older men. However, this procedure may not be acceptable to a high enough proportion of men to make it a useful screening procedure.

Screening tests are not usually sufficiently reliable on their own to make a diagnosis and so a further diagnostic test is also required. For example, if a cervical smear is abnormal this does not make the diagnosis of cervical cancer but, rather, leads on to colposcopy – which is a more definitive test. Similarly, a positive mammogram leads to a biopsy rather than directly to a breast cancer diagnosis. It is important that the diagnostic tests are also acceptable and that they have appropriate sensitivity and specificity – although for a diagnostic test specificity is more important than sensitivity. It is also important that if a population screening programme is commenced it must be continued indefinitely as to offer it to part of the population only, or to offer for only a certain period of time would be inequitable.

Treatment criteria

If a screening programme is commenced the health system should anticipate and allow for the increased rate of the disease that will be picked up if the screening is successful. Thus, for example, to offer breast cancer screening is not appropriate if there are not the resources available to treat the additional cases of early breast cancer that screening will identify. Just as the screening and diagnostic tests must be acceptable to the population, the treatment offered must also be acceptable. This is why, for example, amniocentesis for the detection of fetal abnormalities is not available in Ireland. The treatment offered for women with fetal abnormalities detected by amniocentesis is therapeutic abortion, which is illegal in Ireland.

Economic criteria

The costs of the screening programme and the follow-on costs of diagnostic testing and treatment must be seen as being affordable. The system should be prepared to place sufficient priority on the programme to ensure its continued funding, in spite of other calls on the healthcare budget.

Other points on screening

Screening was originally described in terms of seeking out early stages of particular illnesses. With the developments in epidemiology, predictors of disease have been identified which, although not actually early manifestations of the disease, have been shown to be worth modifying in order to reduce morbidity or mortality. A good example of such a risk factor is hypertension. Hypertension is not a disease per se; it is not even an early manifestation of the diseases for which it serves as a predictor, namely ischaemic heart disease and stroke. However, many studies have now shown that treatment to lower blood pressure reduces morbidity or mortality from these diseases. Hence the screening model can be applied.

If we screen populations for high blood pressure and treat those with blood pressure above certain ranges we can prevent disease. The criteria regarding whether risk factors of this sort are worth seeking out in the population are broadly similar to those described for classical screening for pre-symptomatic disease. However, whether or not a risk factor satisfies the criteria for screen will usually depend on the level set for that risk factor. Thus it is not worth screening for blood pressures close to the normal range but it is increasingly worthwhile screening for higher and higher levels of blood pressure.

Screening programmes often identify people who are positive on the screening test but who go on to prove negative on the diagnostic test. Such patients, who may outnumber those in whom disease is confirmed, may be caused considerable unnecessary anxiety. Furthermore, when screening for a disease is started it naturally engenders a general concern about that particular disease in the population – indeed, if it did not the take-up of screening would be less than desired. Thus, patients who are awaiting screening, and even those who have screened negative, will also have a heightened anxiety. It is difficult to quantify these anxieties and, hence, to make allowance for them in determining whether or not to raise a screening programme. Research on these negative effects of screening is ongoing and it is now accepted that decisions about launching future screening programmes need to take into account the psychological effects of screening on patients who are false positive on the test, and on the population in general.

Lead-time and length bias are two other important issues in judging whether or not screening is worthwhile. Screening tests for a cancer will tend to detect the cancer at an earlier stage than it might otherwise have been seen – patients whose cancer is detected by screening will appear to live longer than those detected by waiting until they present with symptoms. For example, if, say, screening followed by treatment were able to detect breast cancer 7 years before death, whereas the same cancer would not present until 4 years later and result in a fatal outcome regardless of treatment 3 years after that, nothing is gained – even though the screening-detected patient would appear to have gained 4 years of life. This is known as 'lead-time bias'.

Screening tests will also pick up a mixture of fast-growing aggressive tumours that respond poorly to treatment as well as slower-growing tumours that do well regardless of treatment. However, slow-growing tumours have a greater chance of being picked up. For example, over a six-month period of screening, a population with the slow-growing tumour has a good chance of the cancer being detected whereas some fast-growing tumours will be missed. Thus slow-growing tumours will be over-represented in screening-detected cancer and, as they are better prognosis tumours, the appearance may be created that screening is more beneficial than it really is. This is known as 'length bias'. Both lead-time and length bias tend to favour screening even in the absence of benefit. To avoid these problems one needs to look not just at overall reduction in mortality but at cause-specific mortality – comparing similar stage and type cancers.

Current and proposed screening programmes

Table 6.3 lists screening programmes that are generally agreed to be worthwhile and are currently operating in general practice. Several other screening procedures are

Table 6.3
Screening programmes in current use in general practice

Screening procedure/test	Target groups	Disease(s) aimed to prevent/detect early
Heel prick	Neonates	Phenylketonuria, homocystinuria, hypothyroidism, other metabolic problems
Hip examination	Children at birth and 6 weeks	Congenital dislocation of the hip
Child health surveillance	Pre-school children	Early detection of physical and mental disabilities
Antenatal care	Pregnant women	Complications of pregnancy
Cervical cytology screening*	Women of child-bearing age	Cervical carcinoma
Mammography*	Postmenopausal women	Breast cancer
Blood pressure measurement	Middle-aged and older men and women	Stroke and coronary heart disease
Older person assessment	Older people (e.g. over 70 years)	Mobility problems, impairment of hearing and vision, cognitive impairment

*Not yet fully operational on a national basis in the Republic of Ireland (as of 2005).

220

proposed but these are controversial as there is no consensus yet as to whether or not they are worthwhile. Examples include:

- PSA for prostate cancer in middle-aged men
- blood glucose in middle-aged people for diabetes
- faecal occult blood tests or sigmoidoscopy in middle-aged people for colorectal cancer
- DEXA scanning of postmenopausal women for osteoporosis.

In all these cases screening of asymptomatic individuals is proposed. Many of these tests are clearly justified in patients with relevant symptoms – and often in patients with other risk factors such as relevant family history.

Health promotion

Screening is only one means to the more general aim of promoting patient health. It is only one of a whole range of preventive medicine services which include other medical interventions such as immunisation, child health surveillance, antenatal care and so on (see Table 6.6). Health promotion is described in even broader terms than those that encompass screening and conventional medical interventions. Downie (see Further Reading) has described health promotion as having a range of domains, these include:

- preventive health education and lifestyle advice
- preventive health protection
- health education for preventive health protection
- positive health education
- positive health protection
- health education towards positive health protection.

The distinction between these different domains of health promotion can usefully be illustrated in relation to the promotion of child health as shown in Table 6.4. In moving down this list of health promotion activities doctors are less likely to be directly involved, but it is important that doctors

Table 6.4
Different domains of health promotion in relation to children's health

Health promotion domain	Application in relation to child health
Disease prevention	Immunisation
Preventive health education	Health education in schools
Preventive health protection	Water fluoridation to prevent dental caries
Health education for preventive health protection	Advertising campaigns to promote childhood immunisations
Positive health education	General dietary education
Positive health protection	Bans on cigarette advertising
Health education for positive health protection	Campaigning for cycle helmet legislation

are aware of these other methods for promoting health so that they can play their part. In relation to the full range of health promotion activities, doctors can also play a role as citizens or become further involved as active campaigners – and some GPs do. Doctors should at least be seen by patients to be supportive of other health promotion endeavours – for doctors to be seen to be neutral or antagonistic can seriously undermine these efforts.

The Canadian Medical Association divide the health promotion generally advocated by doctors into:

- health enhancement
- risk avoidance
- risk reduction
- early identification of disease, which is equivalent to secondary prevention as is usually described in public health
- reduction in complications, which is equivalent to tertiary prevention as is described in public health.

The use of this categorisation is illustrated in relation to cardiovascular disease in Table 6.5.

Table 6.5
Preventive health strategies for cardiovascular disease

Preventive strategy	Application to cardiovascular disease
Health enhancement	Way to Health (Sli na Slainte in Ireland) – marked out walks signposted and publicised to general public to encourage people to walk more
Risk avoidance	Cigarette advertising bans
Risk reduction	Smoking cessation clinics
Early identification of disease (equivalent to secondary prevention)	Screening for hypertension, hyperlipidaemia, diabetes etc.
Reduction in complications (equivalent to tertiary prevention)	Prescribing of aspirin, beta-blockers, statins etc. for people with established cardiovascular disease and cardiac rehabilitation programmes

Effecting behavioural change

In many health promotion activities, and especially those that involve lifestyle change, a major task of the doctor is to get patients to change their behaviour. There has been a lot of research in health psychology that can inform efforts to persuade patients to modify their lifestyles. An early understanding of people's health-related behaviour came from the Health Belief model (Becker – see Further Reading). According to this model, people's health-related behaviour and their willingness to change behaviour in relation to a health risk is governed by a number of factors that include:

- their perception of the *seriousness* of the illness
- their perception of their own *susceptibility* to the illness (people are very prone to consider that risk factors for illnesses apply to others but not to themselves, as this is an important psychological defence against the anxiety that is provoked by recognising their own vulnerabilities)

- the extent to which they see any *solution* to their health risk as viable.

For example, to tackle a preventive health issue such as the risk of cardiovascular disease arising from cigarette smoking, the doctor must persuade patients that the disease is *serious*, that they are personally *susceptible* to the disease and that a smoking cessation clinic or nicotine replacement therapy is a *solution* that will work for them.

Later work by Prochaska and DiClemente (see Further Reading) has highlighted how people may vary in how ready they are to undertake the complex psychological adjustments that have to be made when overcoming an addictive behaviour such as smoking. Thus, they have constructed a model of behaviour change (the trans-theoretical or stages-of-change model), which highlights how someone may be in one of four states of readiness to change:

- **Pre-contemplation** stage – when people have little or no interest in changing their lifestyle or behaviour.
- **Contemplation** stage – when people are interested in the possibility of change but have not yet 'taken the plunge'.
- **Action** stage – where they are actually in the process of making the change.
- **Maintenance** stage – in which they may be having to struggle to maintain their new lifestyle.

The model also recognises that patients may relapse and go through the different stages several times before fully adopting the new lifestyle.

In order to offer the most appropriate assistance, therefore, the GP needs to determine where on the 'stages of change' the patient currently is. People in the pre-contemplation phase are most likely to be helped by information about the risks associated with their lifestyle but will not be helped by specific guidance on how to give up. Contemplators are greatly helped by advice focussed on the specifics of the giving-up process. People in the action phase, though, need psychological support and encouragement to stick with their action and are not helped with information on risks, for instance. Finally, people in the maintenance phase also need encouragement and support, though perhaps not as intensely as in the action phase.

Implementing this model is by a process called motivational interviewing. This model has been applied to a range of health behaviours such as smoking cessation, alcohol withdrawal and abstinence, dietary modification and so forth.

Nutrition and health

The relationship between nutrition and health is a complex one. Under-nutrition with major dietary components occurs as marasmus or kwashiorkor, while lack of more specific dietary components may occur as specific nutrient deficiency syndromes such as scurvy (vitamin C deficiency). While these conditions are still all too common in the developing world, the more prevalent problems in the developed world are those associated with over-nutrition or nutritional imbalances.

Obesity (defined as excessive accumulation of body fat) is rapidly becoming a major public health issue. It is mainly due to excess dietary intake of energy-rich foods, although reduced physical activity exacerbates the problem. A great variety of health problems are associated with obesity including cardiovascular diseases, diabetes mellitus, various cancers and osteoarthritis.

Lack of particular dietary components or excess of others can also contribute to the risk of other diseases. Cancers and cardiovascular diseases associated with lack of anti-oxidant vitamins (particularly vitamins A, C and E). Lack of dietary fibre may be associated with bowel diseases including diverticular disease and colorectal cancer. Excess dietary salt is known to be associated with hypertension.

What constitutes a 'healthy diet' is now reasonably well defined. Fortunately, there is a good deal of overlap in the diet that is thought to be best to prevent the various conditions on which nutrition has a major influence. Thus the diet that reduces the risk of heart disease is also one that will reduce the risk of diabetes and certain cancers. The features of a healthy diet are listed in Box 6.2.

Box 6.2   Components of a healthy diet

- Low in fat, especially saturated fat (i.e. fat from animal sources)
  - total fat intake should be kept between 20% and 35% of calories and less than 10% of calories should be in the form of saturated fats
  - cholesterol intakes should not exceed 300 mg per day
- Low in salt (less than 6 g per day)
- Carbohydrates mainly in the form of complex carbohydrates
- High in fibre
- High in anti-oxidant vitamins (A, C & E)
  - ideally consumed in the form of fruit and vegetables (5 or more servings per day)
- Alcohol should be kept within recommended limits
  - i.e. 21 units per week for men and 14 units per week for women
- Overall calorie intake should not exceed one's energy needs
  - typically, for adults, this is about 2000 calories per day

There are now a number of educational aids and guides to healthy eating that can be used to assist people adopt these recommendations. One widely used example is the Food Pyramid. Another is the DASH (Dietary Approaches to Stop Hypertension) eating plan, which, while devised specifically for people with hypertension, provides guidance that is applicable to anyone wishing to improve their health through good nutrition. The healthy eating guidelines above are also applicable, with some minor modifications, to people needing to lose weight (who will obviously need to consume fewer calories) and patients with diabetes and other problems.

GPs are often asked by patients for dietary advice – particularly patients concerned about their weight. There are other patients for whom GPs may wish to offer guidance on their food intake because of a specific health problem like diabetes. Offering advice and guidance alone, however, will not usually lead to change of diet or weight-loss. Such advice must be combined with assistance in effecting the necessary behaviour change. Thus, to help patients change to a healthier eating pattern the GP will also need to take them through the stages of change (see above).

Health promotion specific to general practice

Table 6.6 lists a range of preventive and health promoting activities typically undertaken in general practice.

Organisation of preventive care in general practice

There are two basic approaches to the identification of patients for specific health promotion interventions in primary care:

Table 6.6
Preventive health and health promotion activities typically undertaken in general practice/primary care

Preventive activity	Type of prevention	Life stage
Immunisation	Primary	Lifelong but especially early childhood
Child health surveillance	Secondary	Pre-school primarily
Antenatal screening	Secondary	During pregnancy
Family planning services	Primary	During reproductive life
Cervical cytology screening	Secondary	During child bearing years
Breast cancer screening	Secondary	50 years onwards
Blood pressure screening and treatment	Secondary	Middle age onwards
Detection and treatment of lipid disorders	Secondary	Middle age onwards but especially in patients with a history of cardiac disease
Smoking cessation, advice and treatment	Secondary	Lifelong or as long as smoking
Chronic disease management arrangements, e.g. diabetes, asthma, etc.	Tertiary (mostly)	As long as has disease
Prophylactic prescribing	Tertiary prevention (mostly)	Usually lifelong

- case finding
- opportunistic health promotion.

Case finding

This involves identifying 'cases' by the systematic screening of part or all of a population. In countries with a system where the patient registers with a particular doctor or practice for primary care services, individuals for screening can more easily be selected. If the register is maintained electronically, as they often are, the process of identifying and writing to patients in the relevant age and/or sex group is greatly facilitated. A register which holds information on sex and age of the population is called an 'age–sex' register and the summoning of patients in this way is usually referred to as a 'call system'. Once a patient has been seen a note, electronic if appropriate, is made of when they need to be seen again and this can be used to generate 'recall' requests in what would then be referred to as a 'call and recall' system.

Where such registered patient lists are not available, it is still possible to identify patients in need of some preventive health measure by a more general invitation to patients in the relevant category.

Opportunistic health promotion

The case-finding approach does not always sit easily with the philosophy of general practice of offering a holistic, patient-centred service that responds to people's expressed needs. An alternative model proposed for general practice is to offer such preventive services opportunistically. Rather than sending for people who have not seen themselves as needing any medical attention, the opportunity that arises when they present themselves is taken to offer them one or more preventive health measures.

This method of implementing preventive health was first highlighted by Stott and Davis (see Further Reading). They refer to the exceptional potential of consultation to address a wider agenda beyond dealing with the specific health problem brought by the patient. The model, illustrated in Figure 6.1, highlights the fact that when the patient consults,

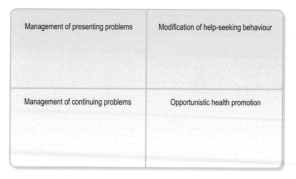

Management of presenting problems	Modification of help-seeking behaviour
Management of continuing problems	Opportunistic health promotion

Fig. 6.1 **The exceptional potential of the GP consultation (after Stott and Davis)**

besides dealing with the presented problem, the GP also has the opportunity to review any continuing health problems the patient might have, the opportunity to educate the patient to use health services more appropriately in future and the opportunity to promote the patient's health.

Opportunistic health promotion has been shown to be an effective approach to child health surveillance and the detection of cardiovascular risk factors. However, if the health promotion activity involves a longer consultation time (as would be the case in an adult health check) this model can prove very difficult to implement during ordinary GP consultations. A variation in the model, proposed by Fuller and Fowler (see Further Reading), is to use the opportunity presented by the patient's attendance to invite the patient to have a more comprehensive health check on another occasion. In the Oxcheck trial of primary health promotion for cardiovascular disease patients were recruited in this opportunistic fashion to a nurse-provided health check. This approach is referred to as 'opportunistic recruitment'.

However cases are identified, further care needs to be properly organised. This can be difficult to accommodate within the normal pattern of surgery visits. Thus, preventive health strategies are often implemented in special clinics (Box 6.3).

Box 6.3   Examples of special clinics for health promotion

- immunisation clinics
- child health and development clinics
- ante-natal clinics
- well-woman clinics
- well-man clinics
- cardiovascular risk assessment clinics
- elderly person surveillance clinic

Further Reading

Becker MH 1974 The health belief model and personal health behaviour. Health Education Monographs vol 2 no 4

Canadian Medical Association 1995 The role of physicians in prevention and health promotion. Canadian Medical Association 153: 208a–d

Downie RS, Tannahill C, Tannahill A 1996 Health promotion: models and values. Oxford University Press, Oxford

Fullard EM, Fowler GH, Gray M 1987 Promoting prevention in primary care: a controlled trial of a low technology, low cost approach. British Medical Journal 294: 1080–1082

Hart CR, Burke P 1992 Screening and surveillance in general practice. Churchill Livingstone, Edinburgh

Imperial Cancer Research Fund OXCHECK Study Group 1995 Effectiveness of health checks conducted by nurses in primary care: final results of the OXCHECK study. BMJ 310: 1099–1104

McWhinney IR 1997 A textbook of family medicine, 2nd edn. Oxford University Press, Oxford

Prochaska JO, DiClemente CC, Norcross JC 1992 In search of how people change – applications to addictive behaviours. American Psychologist 47: 1102–1114

Stephenson A 2003 A textbook of general practice, 2nd edn. Hodder Arnold, Oxford

Stott NCH, Davis RH 1979 The exceptional potential in each primary care consultation. J RoyCollGP 29: 201–205

US Department of Health and Human Services and US Department of Agriculture Dietary Guidelines for Americans 2005

Wilson JMG, Junger G 1968 Principles and practice of screening for disease. World Health Organization: Geneva: (Public Health Papers No 34)

7 Prescribing

Prescribing a medicine is the commonest intervention undertaken by GPs. It is estimated that 50–70% of patients are prescribed something in a consultation with their GP. This also means, though, that a large proportion of patients presenting to their GP are not issued with a prescription. Alternatives to prescribing open to a GP include:

- Do nothing – 'intelligent inactivity'
- Advise patient on non-pharmacological ways of dealing with their problem, e.g. change of lifestyle (diet, exercise, alcohol consumption etc.)
- Counselling or psychologist help

- Encourage home or folk remedies (if safe and appropriate to patient's problem)
- Recommend purchase of an over-the-counter medicine.

Where the patient has a problem that is unlikely to benefit from any kind of medical intervention, 'intelligent inactivity' is the correct response. It may reassure an anxious patient that a problem thought to be very serious is not in fact worthy of serious medical attention.

Non-pharmacological management and encouraging the use of home remedies have the advantage of avoiding medicalisation. The purchase of over-the-counter remedies, besides possibly being cheaper than paying prescription charges (for patients liable for these), empowers patients by increasing their confidence in dealing with minor medical ailments. When a prescription is deemed necessary, information must be provided to the patient along with the written prescription form.

Prescribing decisions

GPs make three distinct types of decisions about prescribing for patients:

- whether or not to prescribe anything
- what to prescribe – drug selection decisions
- when to start using new drugs and when to stop using old drugs.

Whether or not to prescribe

In deciding whether or not to prescribe, prescribers should remain clear about their goals. Possible goals of prescribing are listed in Box 7.1.

Being clear about the aims of therapy at the outset has implications for the duration of treatment. Replacement and prophylactic medicines are usually intended to be taken life-long. Other types of medicines are usually used for a defined course of treatment.

Box 7.1   Goals of prescribing in primary care

The goal of any GP prescription can be to:

- Effect a cure, e.g. antibiotics for pneumonia (surprisingly rare in medical practice)
- Achieve a degree of control over a disease process, e.g. disease-modifying drugs in rheumatoid arthritis
- Replace something missing from the body, e.g. thyroxine to treat hypothyroidism
- Provide preventative measures against such conditions as stroke or heart attack
- Alleviate symptoms, e.g. analgesics used to relieve pain regardless of cause

The goal of therapy also has implications for the extent to which the medicine may be regarded as either essential, desirable or optional. With the passage of time, patients accumulate more and more health problems – and more and more medicines to deal with these. In order to prevent poly-pharmacy (i.e. the prescribing of too many medicines) and the attendant risks of drug interactions, it may become necessary to drop medicines from the patient's regimen. It is much easier to drop less essential medicines if the patient has been informed of the relative importance of each medicine.

Even where drugs are available for the treatment of a patient's problem, non-drug aspects of management should still be considered. Furthermore, although a course of treatment may suggest itself, a doctor's intervention is not always necessary. Self-treatment, with or without self-medication, may still be feasible – and even desirable. It is often better for patients to manage minor ailments themselves – not only does this save on drug costs, whether incurred by patient or state or health system, but it also saves on doctor time. Furthermore, it enables and empowers the patient to manage future occurrences of the condition without resort to medical aid. The disadvantages are that patients may persist with self-management when they might be better seeking medical assistance

233

Education on the safe and effective use of self-treatment and self-medication is an ongoing challenge. Self-treatment may also be supported by advice and information provided by nurses or pharmacists. New primary care structures in the UK are enabling both nurses and pharmacists to become prescribers, in addition to GPs (see also Chapter 10).

Drug selection decisions

If a drug treatment is to be prescribed, it should be the safest, most effective, most appropriate and most economic available. Unfortunately, the selection of the correct drug is not always as simple as this advice suggests. Often there are trade-offs to be made between safety, efficacy, appropriateness and cost (see Fig. 7.1).

Drugs that are the safest are not always the most effective. For example, ibuprofen, rightly regarded as one of the safest non-steroidal anti-inflammatory agents (NSAIDs), is not the most effective. By contrast, indomethacin is a very effective NSAID, but it is more prone than most to causing side effects. The trade-off between safety and efficacy is also apparent within the dosing range of individual drugs. For many drugs a higher dose achieves a greater therapeutic effect – but at the cost of an increased risk of adverse effects.

An appropriate drug is one that is suitable and acceptable to the patient. For example, antibiotic syrups are more appropriate for small children than are tablets or capsules. Slow- or modified-release preparations that allow once daily

234

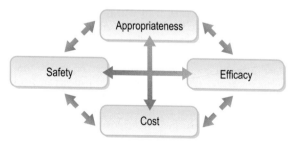

Fig 7.1 **Trade offs involved in drug selection.**

dosing are often more convenient and, arguably, more appropriate for some patients. There may, though, be a trade-off between appropriateness and cost. Drugs with formulations that make them more convenient or acceptable to patients may be more expensive – sometimes much more – than simpler, more traditional formulations.

Trade-offs may also occur between cost and safety or cost and efficacy, and between appropriateness and safety and appropriateness and efficacy – but these are much less common.

Doctors sometimes argue that they should not have to concern themselves with the cost of drugs and that they should be able to choose freely whatever medicine they believe will provide the best balance between safety, efficacy and appropriateness. This is increasingly recognised as unrealistic – healthcare spending is limited, regardless of who is funding it, and money spent on drug costs is very often money that will not be available for other forms of healthcare. This is now being made explicit by healthcare funders, with schemes to make GPs more aware of and responsive to drug costs. In both the UK and Ireland there are drug budgeting schemes in operation, which set a budget for GPs within which they are encouraged to keep their prescribing costs (see also Chapter 12).

In hospital, the arrival of the nurse with the drugs trolley gives the patient little option but to take the medicine prescribed. In the community setting the decision of whether or not to take a medicine ultimately rests with the patient. For this reason, if no other, the doctor should seek to involve the patient in the decision of whether or not a medicine will be prescribed and, indeed, as to what that medicine should be (see also Compliance, below).

Prescribing a drug for the first time

Before starting to use a drug for the first time there are some important considerations for the prescribing doctor. The doctor needs to have some reasonably detailed information about any drug prescribed – the best time to acquire this information is before beginning to use the drug. The GP should know something about:

- the purported mode or modes of action of the drug
- the conditions for which it is indicated and any conditions for which it is contraindicated
- any known adverse effects and which of these are common and/or potentially serious
- the usual dosage and prescribing regimen for the drug
- how this should be modified for any special groups of patients such as children, elderly, patients with renal and/or hepatic impairment.

Drug information sources

Statement of product characteristics/data sheet

It is a legal requirement that the manufacturer or distributor of every medical product produce a statement of the product's characteristics in a standard format. This information, formerly referred to as the data sheet, is the definitive information for prescribers about each drug. In medico-legal cases it may be construed as the knowledge a doctor would be expected to have about any drug prescribed. Statements of product characteristics for most of the medicines available are compiled into a compendium which is supplied free of charge to all GPs.

In the UK, this compendium is compiled by the Association of the British Pharmaceutical Industry and in Ireland it is supplied by the Irish Pharmaceutical Healthcare Association. They are also available on the internet (see Further Reading).

MIMS – The Monthly Index of Medical Specialties

This is a listing of the most commonly prescribed drugs with some brief information about how the drug is presented (i.e. the doses and formulations available), appropriate dosages, major indications, contraindications and adverse effects, and special precautions that should be taken. The production of this pocket-sized manual is supported primarily by the pharmaceutical industry through advertising. The information in it is abbreviated and may not be adequate for the safe prescribing of a drug.

British National Formulary

The British National Formulary is produced by the British Medical Association, the Pharmaceutical Society of Great Britain, and the Department of Health. It is updated twice yearly and is supplied free to all general practitioners in the UK. It is a very convenient and highly regarded source of reliable drug information for prescribers.

Drug and Therapeutics Bulletin

This is a newsletter published bi-monthly by the Consumers' Association which seeks to provide independent advice on therapeutics for doctors. It is sent free of charge to general practitioners in the UK.

Drug company mailings/literature

Pharmaceutical companies supply lots of information on their products to doctors. Advertisements are required to include specified information which is usually an abbreviated version of their statement of product characteristics (see above). While such information is useful, prescribers need to bear in mind that it comes from a source that has a vested interest in promoting the use of the particular product being described.

Word of mouth

As well all the above written information about medicines, GPs gain a good deal of information about new drugs by word of mouth from GP colleagues, from hospital colleagues, from expert speakers at medical meetings and conferences, and from pharmaceutical company representatives.

Clinical trials

The definitive source of information about the efficacy and safety of new drugs is the clinical trials of the drug reported in peer-reviewed medical journals. Prescribing doctors should be aware of the features of a clinical trial that make its results more or less worth relying on in clinical practice.

Assessing the scientific evidence is one of the key elements of the evidence-based medicine philosophy. A full description of the evidence-based medicine approach to the assessment of clinical trials is beyond the scope of this book – interested readers are referred to an appropriate text on evidence-based medicine. However, there are a few key questions of a clinical trial that all prescribers should ask:

- was assignment of patients to treatment random?
- were all patients who entered the trial accounted for at the end? (i.e. was there an intention-to-treat analysis done)
- do results apply in your patient(s)?

See Table 7.1 for a comparison of all these drug-information sources.

Information as part of the prescription

It is important that patients are given enough information about their medicines to ensure they use them safely and appropriately. Box 7.2 contains a suggested minimum information set that should be given to patients when prescribing them a drug, particularly when prescribing it for the first time.

Alternatives to prescribing

These have been described as the 'larder' the 'blackboard' and the 'doctor'.

- The *larder* refers to the fact that there are many remedies suitable for the relief of symptoms of minor ailments that are available in the home. Honey and

Table 7.1
Advantages and disadvantages of different drug information sources

Drug information source	Advantages	Disadvantages
Manufacturer's statement of product characteristics	Comprehensive information on every drug Sets the (medico-legal) standard of drug information a doctor is expected to have about each medicine prescribed Predictable lay-out of information on each drug Supplied free by manufacturer – available annually/ biannually in compendium supplied free to all GPs	Very detailed (maybe too detailed) Every possible adverse effect listed, mainly to defend manufacturer
MIMS (Monthly Index of Medical Specialities)	Brief information on all most-commonly used drugs Up to date information on drug costs (wholesale price given) Good for identifying brand names of drugs Information on shape, colour and markings on tables – useful for identification Brief prescribing advice at beginning of each section Some useful tables comparing drugs included Updated monthly (White coat) pocket sized Supplied free to prescribers	Information very limited Safety information (in particular) incomplete Comparative information very scant Supported by pharmaceutical industry – cannot be regarded as independent opinion Bulges with advertising
British National Formulary	Brief information on most-commonly used drugs – slightly more detail than MIMS Independently produced More specific in recommending some drugs over others	Limited information, especially on drugs it does not recommend Not comprehensive in identifying all brands of some medicines

239

Table 7.1 Continued.

Drug information source	Advantages	Disadvantages
	Identifies drugs of limited value	Difficult to access relevant information from this source during a consultation
	Lots of additional information on interactions, drugs in pregnancy, drugs in breast milk etc.	Not always able to comment on drug before GPs begin to use it
	Includes information on costs	Relatively long articles (compared to BNF, MIMS)
	(White coat) pocket sized	Considered by some to be 'too opinionated'
	Updated 6 monthly	Not independent
	Supplied free to all prescribing doctors (in UK only)	Over-emphasis on efficacy and underplaying of disadvantages of products
	Available free on the internet www.bnf.org	Not always reliable
Drug and Therapeutics Bulletin	Independent and carefully vetted drug information	Can be biased in hidden ways
	Very good for placing drugs in the therapeutic armamentarium	Not always accessible (may be published in a huge variety of biomedical periodicals)
	Good overviews of therapeutic areas	Difficult for ordinary GP to interpret
	Good coverage of new drugs as they come along	
	Supplied free to all GPs (UK)	
	Well written – succinct yet not too formulaic or dry	
Drug company literature	Well produced – glossy, attractive to look at and handle	
	Has the key information to enable prescribing – dosages, regimen, etc.	
	Readily available (difficult to avoid)	
	Very convenient	
Word of mouth from peers and experts	Can be interrogated on specific points about the medicine (interactive)	
Reports of clinical trials (and other research)	The definitive source of drug safety and efficacy information	
	Does not answer all the questions needed for clinical use	

Box 7.2 **Proposed minimum information set about drugs prescribed for patients**

- The name of the drug or drugs – this should, ideally, be both the brand name and the generic name but one of these as a minimum
- What the drug is supposed to do
- How and when they are to be taken
- How long they are to be taken for
- Common adverse effects and interactions the patient should look out for
- The extent to which the medicines are thought, by the doctor, to be essential to health

lemon for coughs and bicarbonate of soda for indigestion are but two examples.

- The *blackboard* refers to the fact that educating the patient about how to self-manage the problem may be more appropriate than issuing a prescription.
- The *doctor* refers to the fact that contact with an attentive and caring doctor can, of itself, be therapeutic and may obviate the need for any formal therapy or prescription.

Misuse of prescription drugs

241

All doctors need to be aware of the potential for drugs to be misused. Some drugs, notably psychotropic drugs, are widely misused and are traded within the drug misusing community so that they acquire a 'street value'. Awareness of this danger should alert doctors to the need to evaluate this risk – both in relation to the drug being selected and the patient for whom it is being prescribed. The GP will generally have knowledge of each patient, allowing reasonably valid judgements to be made of whether or not a patient is trustworthy in this regard.

Doctors need to be particularly wary of patients who are not well known to them demanding prescriptions for drugs with a street value or a potential for misuse.

Non-compliance or non-adherence

One of the major problems facing doctors is that patients do not always take their medicines as prescribed. This problem was traditionally referred to as 'non-compliance', although the term 'non-adherence' is rather less pejorative and is now the preferred term. Research into non-adherence has found that:

- one-third of patients take their drugs as prescribed
- one-third of patients take their drugs but not exactly as prescribed
- one-third does not take the drugs at all.

However, the extent to which strict adherence to the doctor's orders is necessary for the therapeutic effect varies. Some drugs are said to be more 'forgiving' than others. Given variable levels of forgiveness from different drugs, we can anticipate that about half the time patient adherence is sufficient to gain therapeutic benefit and the other half of the time adherence is insufficient to gain therapeutic benefit.

Adherence varies with a great number of other factors – knowledge of these can allow strategies to be adopted by doctors to minimise non-adherence. Adherence depends on the patient understanding and following the doctor's instructions. Non-adherence is, therefore, more likely if:

- the medication regimen is too complex
- the patient is elderly
- the patient has difficulties understanding the doctor, e.g. language difficulties.

Ways of reducing non-adherence include:

- using simpler dosing regimens – once or twice daily schedules are much more likely to be followed properly than those involving more frequent dosing
- repeating instructions
- checking the patient's understanding of instructions before he or she leaves
- backing up verbal instructions with corresponding written instructions.

It is surprising to doctors to realise that, sometimes, patients deliberately do not take their medicines as prescribed. This is referred to as 'intentional non-adherence'. This may relate to the patient being generally disinclined to take any medicines (referred to as being 'drug averse') or it may be because the patient has specific reservations about the particular treatment proposed. These reservations may arise from a reluctance of the patient to accept that they are even ill in the first place or it may arise from concerns about the possible ill effects of the medicines – such concerns are not always misplaced. It may also relate to a lack of trust or faith in the prescribing doctor.

Intentional non-adherence may be reduced by adopting an open approach with patients, exploring their broader concerns about their condition and about the treatment in particular. It may also be that intentional non-adherence cannot be eradicated but, in dialogue with patients, a better mutual understanding between doctor (as to what is desirable) and patient (as to what is acceptable) can be arrived at. This is the aim behind the movement promoting 'concordance'. Concordance is not a new term for compliance or adherence, but rather it is recognition that the treatment course that will be followed by the patient will usually be the one the patient agrees with and so efforts should be directed at obtaining such an agreement.

Practical prescribing

Writing a prescription

Prescriptions should be written on either a special form for the public health services (FP10 in the UK and GMS Prescription form in Ireland) or on notepaper with the doctor's name and address if it is for private patients. The prescription should contain the patient's name and address and, for children under 12, their age or date of birth. For each drug prescribed, the name of the drug (either generic or brand name) should be clearly written followed by:

- the dosage
- the dosing regimen (i.e. once daily, twice daily, 4-hourly etc.)

- the total amount of medicine to be supplied as either total quantity of medicine or as the number of days of treatment to be dispensed.

Prescriptions *must* be signed and dated by the prescriber.

The amount prescribed on NHS (UK) or GMS (Ireland) forms is usually expected to represent a maximum of one month's supply with a few exceptions (e.g. the contraceptive pill in the UK). Private prescriptions may contain a note of how many times the course of treatment specified can be redispensed without a medical consultation.

Controlled drugs

Controlled drugs are those where prescribing and dispensing is subject to tighter regulation and additional requirements over and above those governing prescription medicines in general. Examples of controlled drugs are opiates and certain benzodiazepines. Controls are usually put in place because of the risk of illicit use of the drug for 'recreational' purposes and/or because of their potential to cause addiction. Where the medicine being prescribed is a controlled drug, the prescription should be *hand written* by the prescribing doctor and the *total dosage to be dispensed must be written in numbers and words*.

Repeat prescribing

Patients with chronic illnesses, patients on replacement therapies such as thyroxine, and patients on various preventive therapies such as anti-hypertensives all need to take their medicine continuously over long periods – most usually for the rest of their lives. Patients need to be monitored while on these medicines. They may need to have their disease or risk status checked periodically and they may need to be monitored for possible adverse effects of their medicines. Being checked regularly also encourages adherence to their medication regimen, as does the opportunity to share their concerns and experiences of living with their illness and their medicine. The frequency of these reviews, though, should be tailored to the patient and the needs of the illness and monitoring programme.

When a prescription is issued for the first time or for episodic illnesses they are usually issued for a maximum of one month's treatment. This is specifically encouraged by the regulations prevailing in the NHS in the UK and the GMS in Ireland. For people on long-term prescriptions monthly review would usually be too frequent – arrangements must be made for them to have repeat prescriptions that can be dispensed at monthly intervals between clinical reviews, without the need for face-to-face contact with their doctor. Such arrangements are beneficial to both doctor and patient – sparing them both the time and inconvenience of more contacts than are clinically necessary.

Thus most practices have administrative arrangements whereby patients can request further supplies of their medicines to be prescribed between their periodic clinical reviews. These administrative arrangements have been greatly facilitated by the advent of practice computerisation such that now up to 75% of prescribing may be occurring via repeat prescribing. However, there are major problems with repeat prescribing systems as they can allow situations to develop whereby patients are continuing to receive their medicines or may be failing to get their medicines without adequate supervision or monitoring.

Research has shown that problems can arise in the administration of the repeat prescribing system, in the management of the system, or in the clinical supervision of the system. A good repeat prescribing system needs to be sufficiently flexible to meet each patient's need for convenience while still being sufficiently tight as to pick up and deal with problems that may arise. The design, setting-up and running of a good repeat prescribing system needs investment of time and effort on the part of all members of the practice team.

Economic aspects

As noted above (see 'Drug selection decisions'), doctors should prescribe the least costly drug that will treat the patient safely and adequately. If they prescribe unnecessarily expensive medicines, the cost of meeting these will have to come out of the resources available to treat other patients. Resources are always limited – those expended in one area are no longer available for expenditure in another. This is a concept in economics known as 'opportunity cost' (see also Chapter 12). However, it is not the absolute cost of medicines that should determine whether or not they are economically appropriate to use, but rather their cost-effectiveness, i.e. how much cost is incurred per unit of health gain.

The relative value of different prescribing strategies can be established using techniques of health economic evaluation. Four basic types of health economic evaluation are available to compare different drugs or prescribing strategies. These are summarised in Table 7.2.

Table 7.2
Different types of health economic evaluations

Type of study	Unit of measurement of outcome	Comments
Cost minimisation study	None	Simple comparison of relative costs regardless of outcome
Cost–benefit study	Monetary units	Benefits are translated into monetary terms to allow comparison with costs
Cost effectiveness study	Natural units (usually relating to illness) – same in all comparator groups, e.g. number of lives saved	Only works where there is sufficient similarity of outcome in different study groups
Cost utility analysis	QALYs (quality of adjusted life years)	Artificial unit relating to quality of life derived to allow comparison between very different health outcomes and relative costs

Over-the-counter medicines and self-medication

Medicines in the UK and Ireland are licensed in three broad categories:

- prescription-only medicines (POMs)
- pharmacy-only medicines (Ps)
- general sales list (GSL) medicines.

POMs can only be dispensed by pharmacists by direction of a doctor's prescription. P medicines are only available through pharmacies but do not require a doctor's prescription. GSL medicines can be bought in a range of outlets including supermarkets, garages and so on. P and GSL medicines, known collectively as over-the-counter medicines (OTCs), are sold to patients who have decided themselves what is ailing them and have opted for an OTC to self-treat.

As time goes by an increasing number of medicines are being relicensed from the POM to the P category and from the P to the GSL category – thereby increasing the scope for patients to self-treat for minor ailments without recourse to doctors. This self-medication can generally be welcomed by doctors because it enables patients to become increasingly self-reliant in managing their own health problems, providing it is not seen as a substitute for consulting a doctor.

In the UK patients can now have certain medicines prescribed by nurses and pharmacists, under new arrangements for primary care being introduced.

247

Further Reading

Harris C 1996 Prescribing in general practice. Radcliffe Medical Press, Oxford

Hobbs R, Bradley C 1998 Prescribing in primary care. Oxford University Press, Oxford

Mant A 1999 Thinking about prescribing: a handbook for quality use of medicines. McGraw Hill, New York

Sackett D, Richardson W, Rosenberg W, Haynes R 1997 Evidence-based medicine: how to practice and teach EBM. Churchill Livingstone, Edinburgh

www.emc.medicines.org.uk (for medicines used in the UK)

www.medicines.ie (for medicines used in Ireland)

Referral to specialists

The vast majority of patients' problems presenting to general practitioners are dealt with by the GP. However, there are occasions when the problem is, or seems to be, beyond the capacity of the GP – who will then seek the help of a specialist colleague by the process of 'referring the patient'. On average only about 5% of patients seen in general practice will be referred but this rate varies widely (see below). As care by specialists usually involves much more complex, expensive and riskier investigations and treatments, there are major clinical, economic and ethical consequences incurred when a decision is made by a GP to refer a patient to a specialist.

Reasons for referral

Reasons for referral by GPs to specialists may be instrumental (i.e. to achieve a straightforward clinical objective) or for

> Box 8.1   Instrumental reasons for GP referral to specialist colleagues
>
> - Diagnosis – when this cannot be achieved by the GP
> - Investigation – especially for tests not available to the GP
> - Treatment – e.g. surgical treatment, chemotherapy and other treatments that cannot be undertaken by the GP
> - Advice on the best treatment or additional management that might be tried by the GP to improve results for the patient
> - Advice on prognosis
> - Second opinion on diagnosis, management, or prognosis or any combination thereof
> - Reassurance of the patient

more subtle reasons not so closely related to obvious clinical goals. Instrumental reasons are listed in Box 8.1, other reasons for referral may include:

- a desire on the part of the GP to share the burden of caring for a patient with a specialist, especially for difficult or demanding patients
- to maintain the doctor–patient relationship
- pressure (or perceived pressure) from the patient or relatives for a referral
- concern about malpractice litigation if a specialist is not involved.

These sorts of reasons for referral may be viewed by GP, specialist or patient as less legitimate and so may not always be communicated to the specialist. However, failure to communicate the real reason for a referral can lead to misunderstandings between specialist, GP and patients as to what is expected from a referral. One large study in England looked at the distribution of these reasons across a sample of 18 754 referrals. It found that, in relation to the principle reason for referral:

- 28% were to establish the diagnosis
- 7% for a specified investigation
- 35% were for a particular treatment or operation

- 14% were for advice on management
- 9% were for the specialist to take over management
- 2% were seeking reassurance that the GP had done all that was required
- 2% were to reassure patients and their families that the GP had done all that was required
- 2% were for other reasons.

Referral rates

Doctors differ widely in the proportions of patients they refer for specialist opinion, advice, diagnosis or treatment. The UK average is reported as being between 4% and 6% of patients consulting or between 10% and 12% of patients registered on the practice list per year. However, in one large study of urban general practice, the range was from 1% to 24% of patients consulting. Table 8.1 shows the proportions referred to different specialties in this urban study. Within these averages there were great variations in proportions referred to different specialties by different GPs and practices.

Table 8.1
Distribution of referrals between selected specialties in a large study of UK urban general practice

251

Specialty	Percentage of referrals
General surgery	18%
General medicine	10%
Gynaecology	10%
ENT	9%
Orthopaedics	10%
Ophthalmology	5%
Dermatology	5%
Paediatrics	4%
Geriatric medicine	2%
Psychiatry	4%

From Wilkin D, Metcalfe D, Leavey R Routledge, London. Anatomy of urban general practice.

Referral rates also vary between different countries, as shown in data derived from the European Referrals Study – a study of 45000 referrals in 15 different countries undertaken in the late 1980s (Table 8.2). Factors influencing referral rates can be classified as:

● patient variables
● provider variables
● healthcare system variables.

Patient variables

Patient variables include age, sex, morbidity, social class. Older patients and female patients are generally referred more often. Female patients are referred more often than males, even when allowance is made for their needs relating to their reproductive function, but it is commensurate with the tendency for women to consult GPs more often than

Table 8.2
Referral rates for different European countries

Country	Referral rate (per 100 consultations)
Norway	8.2
Italy	6.7
Denmark	6.6
Yugoslavia*	6.4
Portugal	5.8
Germany (former West Germany)**	5.6
Spain	5.5
United Kingdom	4.7
Netherlands	4.5
Republic of Ireland	4.2
Germany (former East Germany)**	4.1
Belgium	3.9
Switzerland	3.8
Hungary	3.5
France	3.4

*The survey was conducted before the dissolution of the former Yugoslavia.
**The survey was conducted before the reunification of Germany.
From RCGP European Referrals Study.

men. Rates of referral vary dramatically depending on the type of conditions being seen. Thus in the Third National Morbidity study (see Government Statistical Service), 2.4% of respiratory conditions seen were referred compared with 33% of patients consulting for neoplasms.

However, in many studies of GP referrals differences in the cases being seen (case mix) are much less than difference seen in referral rates of different doctors. This indicates that doctor factors are, perhaps, more important than case mix in accounting for variations in referral rates. The effect of social class is much less consistent and may be accounted for to some extent by differences in consulting rates by different social class and differences in morbidity by social class. When these factors are controlled for, differences in referral by social class tend to diminish or disappear.

Provider variables

Differences in the knowledge and/or experience of doctors have most commonly been mooted as explanations for variations in referral rates. Younger, less experienced doctors are often thought to be more prone to refer their patients, but this has not been supported consistently by research. Similarly, although it has been proposed that doctors with greater knowledge of a clinical sub-specialty might need to refer less often to that specialty, the evidence more often points to the opposite, i.e. that doctors with more knowledge of a specialty refer to it more often. Overall, though, the literature indicates no consistent relationship to differences in specialist knowledge between GPs.

Likewise, membership of a college of general practice or additional diplomas or qualifications do not seem to correlate with higher or lower referral rates. However, the inability to demonstrate clear relationships between provider characteristics and referral rates may be more to do with an inability to identify and measure the relevant characteristics than with any lack of importance of these variables in explaining variations in referral rates.

Some GPs working within the same practice when dealing with very similar cases can still vary considerably in their referral rates. This has led to the suggestion that each GP

253

has a unique 'referral threshold'. This seems likely to relate more to attitudes to risk, tolerance of uncertainty and other psychological variables affecting clinical decision-making than to GP variables such as experience or knowledge.

Dowie's study (see Further Reading) of GP referrals identified important aspects of the cognitive processes of GPs that could possibly account for differences in referral behaviour. She found that, as well as having different levels of knowledge, they had variable reliance on information provided by investigations. GPs also attached importance to their esteem in the eyes of specialist colleagues, which was a factor they considered in their decisions to refer or not. Dowie's model relates only to referrals for diagnosis of potentially acute serious illness.

A more refined, all-encompassing model has been proposed by Wilkin and Smith (Box 8.2). The importance of both models is that they focus attention on the thought processes of referring doctors, while taking into account the emotional context in which decisions are made (Fig. 8.1).

Box 8.2 Wilkin & Smith's model for referral decisions*

In this model GPs are considered to make a series of judgements about whether:

- they have enough information to deal adequately with the patient's problem
- there are risks to the patient in not referring
- there are risks to the doctor's esteem in the eyes of colleagues if they do refer
- the GP can generate an adequate diagnosis or management plan themselves
- a better diagnosis or management would be achieved by referral
- the benefits of referral outweigh the costs when compared to alternatives

*From Wilkin & Smith 1987 Explaining variation in GP referrals to hospital. Family Practice 4:160–169, with permission.

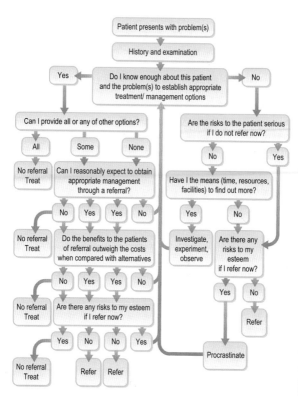

Fig. 8.1 Model of the referral decision (from Wilkin & Smith 1987 Explaining variation in GP referrals to hospital. Family Practice 4:160–169, with permission)

Healthcare system variables

Other variables that may impinge on referral patterns relate to the healthcare system itself. For instance the availability and accessibility of hospital services may affect GPs referral decisions. It has been shown that the number of outpatients seen in certain specialties is strongly associated with the provision of consultants in those specialties. In urban areas proximity to the hospital does not seem to be a major determinant of referral rates but distance from the nearest hospital in rural areas is likely to affect referral rates. There are marked differences between overall referral rates between rural and urban areas – though the differences between the referral rates of different GPs are always larger than these other variables.

Differences in referral patterns between different countries are much more substantial than any of these intra-country differences. In a very large study of referral patterns in 15 different countries in the 1980s the range of average referral rates was found to vary from less than 4% to nearly 7%. There were also considerable differences observed between countries in what actually constituted a referral, the financial and other incentives and disincentives that existed for doctors to refer or not refer, and the extent to which patients could influence the referral decisions of their doctor or refer themselves to a specialist without consulting a GP.

Thus, in some countries there is a substantial proportion of what are called 'indirect referrals' where the GP refers a patient to a specialist but without actually having seen the patient. This may relate to the payment system that may require validation by a GP for a patient to see or continue seeing a specialist. In some countries GPs compete commercially with specialists (see the GP gatekeeper role, below) who may provide general as well as specialist care. In this case there is a disincentive to the GP to refer for fear of losing the patient. In other countries there may be financial incentives to GPs or to patients that encourage GPs to refer more of their patients or patients to demand more referrals. Thus, for example, if the health insurance system refunds specialist care but not general practitioner care, the GP will be under more pressure to refer a greater proportion of patients.

Inappropriate or excessive referral

While it is difficult to determine an optimum referral rate, it is clear that too many and too few referrals from general practice to hospital are both undesirable. If too many patients are referred from general practice both the GP and the specialist run the danger of becoming deskilled:

- the GP suffers lost opportunity to hone skills on patients
- the specialist's skills are diluted by less severe cases or cases that did not need specialist skills – leading to a smaller proportion of cases where skills can be honed.

Also, if patients are referred too readily they run the danger of being inappropriately labelled as having a serious condition when they do not. However, a GP who is too reluctant to refer patients exposes them to a different range of dangers. The patient denied timely diagnosis:

- may suffer unnecessarily
- may deteriorate to the point where treatment is more difficult, costly, painful or possibly even futile – i.e. beyond the point at which treatment is effective
- may be denied a better treatment which is only available through hospital.

GPs learn from the patients they refer about what is regarded by specialists as the most modern (and presumably most effective) treatment available. A GP who goes for a long time without this contact with hospital medicine may become out-of-date in the approach to or management of patient problems.

Appropriate referral

Given the possibility of both under- and over-referral, referrals may be classified as either appropriate or inappropriate. However, this begs the question of to whom it is appropriate. Patients, GPs and specialists may all differ in what they consider to be an appropriate referral. A patient with chest pain who is worried that there might be a cardiac problem may well view referral to a cardiologist as appropriate –

whereas the cardiologist, recognising it as a case of costo-chondritis, may view the visit as a waste of expertise. Likewise, a GP seeing a patient with psoriasis may refer the patient to a dermatologist in order to access ultraviolet therapy. The dermatologist, however, might not consider this treatment necessary and may view the referral as inappropriate. The judgement of appropriateness depends on the doctor's position in the process. However, all referrals that are worthwhile should be associated with some perceptible health or social gain.

Furthermore, knowing that a patient does not have a disease may be associated with important health and/or social gain. Likewise, referral at a very early stage of a disease – or even when there are only risk factors for a disease – may still be worthwhile because there may be prevention of future health loss. An example of this might be referral of a family member for bowel investigations when one of the family is found to have familial polyposis coli.

Referrals, therefore, may be judged in terms of the health or social gains available. In this regard, there can be said to be three categories of referral:

- referrals which virtually everyone would agree should be made, e.g. a patient with symptoms strongly suggestive of a malignancy
- referrals which virtually everyone would agree are unnecessary, such as referral of a young otherwise fit adult for symptoms suggestive of a common cold
- referrals where it is a matter of judgement as to whether referral is worthwhile and/or timely.

It is in relation to this last judgement that individual doctors seem to have a referral threshold such that, when their anxiety about the balance of risks between referral and not referring swing in favour of referral, they will refer. This may vary from doctor to doctor and may vary from one clinical area to another according to the doctors' confidence in dealing with certain health problems – and possibly their training in that specialty area.

Referral guidelines

One means of trying to reduce variability in referrals between GPs, and ensuring more appropriate referrals, is through the development of guidelines. Guidelines have been devised for most common clinical problems and specific guidance on when patients should be referred to secondary care is often incorporated within these (see also Chapter 5). The production, dissemination and implementation of guidelines, however, is a complex, costly and sometimes very difficult process. Providing useful guidance on referral is particularly difficult. Guidance may be either so self-evident as to be hardly worth stating, or so general as to be of little practical use. On the other hand, very specific guidance may only be able to cover a minority of clinical scenarios.

It has been shown that guidelines can be effective in changing physician behaviour, including referral behaviour – but only if the guidelines are effectively disseminated and implemented. This requires that local practising clinicians have a say in the development of the guidelines, that multiple methods of dissemination through specific educational programmes are used, and that implementation is undertaken in conjunction with some form of patient-specific reminders or prompts for doctors. Even with effective dissemination and implementation strategies it has, so far, been difficult to prove the cost-effectiveness of guideline development in all but a few instances. Work on how to develop effective guidelines is continuing.

The GP as gatekeeper

In some countries, including the UK and Ireland, a patient can generally only be seen following referral by a GP. In other countries patients may be referred to specialists by GPs or family doctors, but are also equally at liberty to seek specialist care themselves and to attend any specialist of their own choosing. Where access to specialists is controlled and restricted to referral via a GP, the GP is said to be acting as a 'gatekeeper'.

Advantages of GPs as gatekeepers
For GPs:

- it enables them to keep track of all the patients' problems and to be kept abreast of the patients' conditions and their diagnosis and treatment
- it is more satisfying for GPs to hold onto patients to manage themselves
- it is a stimulus to continuing professional development.

For specialists:

- it allows them to maintain their special skills without having these diluted by dealing with larger numbers of people with little or no illness
- it ensures that these skills are used to best effect
- it avoids specialists having to deal with other problems where they may be lacking expertise.

For patients:

- it avoids patients having to judge their own condition and decide if it requires a specialist
- it avoids having to choose which specialist to attend
- it avoids the risks attendant on getting either of these decisions wrong
- it may avoid undue expense (specialists generally charge more than generalists regardless of the nature of the problem ultimately diagnosed).

For the healthcare system:

- it should lead to the most effective use of resources – both specialist and GP
- it certainly helps contain healthcare costs
- it can lead to better health outcomes overall.

Disadvantages of GPs as gatekeepers
For GPs:

- it places all the responsibility for the referral decisions on them
- it may lead to them coming under pressure from the health payment system to restrict access to expensive specialists
- it may lead to pressure from patients to refer to specialists that the GP does not see as appropriate.

For specialists:

- it may mean that patients they would like to see, possibly at an early stage of their illness, may not be seen because they have not got past the GP gatekeeper
- it may be seen by some specialists as a restriction on their practice (or earning capacity).

For patients:

- it can also be perceived as a restriction on their choice of healthcare provision
- it can lead to worse outcomes if the gate is too restrictive.

For the healthcare system:

- it can negate the usual effects of market forces of competition helping contain healthcare costs (as both specialists and GPs may be able to charge the system more for their services)
- it can be more difficult to administer
- it may be unpopular with patients, which will make it politically unattractive to a democratically elected administration.

261

Referral and discharge letters

The usual mode of making a referral is by means of a referral letter from the GP to the specialist. The ideal referral letter should highlight the points listed in Box 8.3. Not all

Box 8.3 The referral letter

The ideal referral letter should highlight:

- name, address, d.o.b. (age) of patient
- presenting complaint/problem
- history of presenting complaint
- past medical history including management of pre-existing problems
- current and past medication(s)
- allergies (if any)
- social history including details of social circumstances and availability or otherwise of non-professional carers
- findings on examination
- results of any investigations
- the referring doctor's opinion of problem/diagnosis
- reason for referral and some indication of perceived urgency
- any specific information/service needed from specialist and the GPs expectation regarding follow up and future care

the items of information will be required on every occasion, though details of the presenting problems and the reason for referral will virtually always be essential.

The referral letter is part of a two-way communication process and there are important requirements of the letters specialists should send to GPs. This most commonly comes in the form of discharge letter, either from an inpatient stay or from an outpatient visit or series of visits. The following information should be considered for inclusion in letters to GPs:

- summary of symptoms
- examination findings
- results of investigations
- diagnosis or summary of problem(s)
- management plan
- nature and quantity of drugs issued
- information given to patient and/or relatives

- follow-up arrangements
- advice on future management.

Again, not all of this information is relevant in every case but several studies of letters from specialists to GPs have found them to be inadequate from the GP's perspective, omitting important items of information. On the other hand, GPs often require information from hospitals about their patients much more quickly than they receive it – a small amount of information received in a timely way is often more useful than a detailed report many weeks later. The best of both worlds for a GP is possibly a brief letter, possibly on a standardised discharge form, followed by a fuller report a little later.

Performance review

All clinicians should be constantly on the look out for ways to judge and enhance the effectiveness of their clinical performance. The most usual process of doing this is known as 'medical audit', in which the care of a group of patients is compared to pre-determined standards as laid down in the literature or in clinical guidelines (see also Chapter 5).

Patients who have been referred are an ideal group to look at with regard to determining the quality of their care. Firstly, they are an easily identifiable group whose care is generally reflected in a fairly clear and detailed way in the referral correspondence and specialist replies. Furthermore, they are clearly an important group who are very likely to have significant clinical problems, whose outcomes will be affected by the quality of care provided.

Looking at referred patients may provide lessons regarding either their primary or secondary care, or both. It will also expose the effectiveness or otherwise of the operation of the primary/secondary care interface. The desire to conduct audit in this area should bring up a discussion of referral criteria that should be used and standards that should be applied. This effort alone is likely to improve the quality of subsequent referrals.

Alternatives to referral

As well as a formal outpatient referral to specialists, GPs have a number of alternative ways of seeking specialist assistance, many of which are under-utilised, including:

- a telephone call to specialists
- domiciliary visits by a specialist
- specialist outreach clinics
- telemedicine
- inter-referral to another GP.

Seeking telephone advice from specialist colleagues should be considered when there is a limited question, such as whether or when to instigate a particular treatment in a patient. It is also useful as a follow-up technique when the specialist has already been involved in the care of the patient and has a record (and possibly a memory) of the particular patient.

A visit by a specialist to a patient in their own home is an alternative that is available almost uniquely in the UK. Traditionally, the GP would also be in attendance to confer with the specialist at the patient's bedside. Nowadays the GP is not usually present and this provision is restricted to fewer specialties such as care of the elderly.

Specialist outreach clinics, where consultants come to the GP's surgery to see patients, have become more feasible as GP practices get larger and so can generate the numbers of referrals to justify the attendance of a specialist on a regular basis. A reasonably widespread example of this approach is liaison psychiatry. Community outreach of specialist services can also be extended to acutely ill patients, who might otherwise need a hospital admission, through so-called 'hospital at home' schemes. This model has also been successfully piloted in the psychiatry area.

Modern IT and telecommunications technology are also beginning to enable the development of telemedicine, whereby expert opinion can be provided to GPs regarding patients without the need for the patient to attend the specialist – who can be a considerable distance away but linked by telephone or video conference. Many GPs now also have specialist skills that are increasingly availed of by colleagues who seek their opinion before, or instead of, referring patients to hospital. This referral from GP to GP is referred to as 'inter-referral'.

Post-discharge and follow-up

The care of patients following referral varies greatly depending on the nature of the problem, the care required and the capacities of both GPs and specialists. For some conditions, such as cancer, a considerable amount of care will be received from the specialist services for quite a long time following initial referral. For other conditions, such as acute appendicitis, virtually all of the care required will be delivered during the hospital admission and all the aftercare can be undertaken in general practice – with a provision for re-referral should unexpected or unusual complications develop.

When primary care provision was fairly primitive, there was a strong tendency for specialists to retain control of the patient's care until a complete recovery took place, or for the rest of the patient's life in the case of chronic diseases. However, as more patients are living longer with one or more chronic diseases, as medical technology becomes simpler to apply in non-hospital settings, and as primary care facilities and capacity improves, more long-term care and follow-up can take place outside hospitals.

A good example is in the area of diabetes care. Historically, once diagnosed with diabetes a patient came under the long-term follow-up of a hospital specialist who undertook all routine patient review, as well as dealing with any crises or complications that arose. In the early 1970s there were attempts to relocate the long-term care of patients with diabetes to general practice settings. These initial attempts were unsuccessful – but this was due to inadequate preparation of general practice for this task. With time, GPs became better equipped, in terms of both infrastructure and training, to manage diabetes care in conjunction with hospitals through various 'shared care' arrangements. Now many patients while perhaps nominally under such a shared care arrangement are effectively looked after almost entirely in general practice. The outcomes from such care can be shown to at least match those achieved by exclusively hospital-based care.

Further Reading

Balint M 1957 The doctor, his patient and the illness. Tavistock Publications, London

Dowie R 1983 General practitioners and consultants: a study of outpatient referrals. The Kings Fund, London

Roland M, Coulter A 1992 Hospital referrals. Oxford University Press, Oxford

Royal College of General Practitioners 1992 The European Study of Referrals from Primary to Secondary Care. Occasional Paper 56. Royal College of General Practitioners, London

Government Statistical Service 1986 Morbidity statistics from general practice 1981–1982: third national study. Her Majesty's Stationery Office

Wilkin D, Hallam L, Leavey R, Metcalfe 1987 Anatomy of urban general practice (particularly Chapter 7, Patterns of Care). Tavistock Publications, London

Doctor–patient communication

The consultation

The meeting between a doctor and a patient is central to the practice of medicine. It is the process by which most health problems are assessed and managed. Encounters that go wrong or are dysfunctional are a significant source of medical error that may have serious clinical and/or economic consequences. In general practice the consultation is particularly crucial – GPs do not have as ready access to the investigative tools available in other medical settings, nor do they have the same opportunities to keep patients under close supervision.

GPs in the UK and Ireland conduct over a million consultations per day and, while they may generally succeed in their consultations with patients, there are problems in communication – as is manifest from the observations in Box 9.1 from research in this area.

Box 9.1   Selection of observations from research into GP communication

- two-thirds of psychological and psychiatric problems presenting to GPs are missed
- 54% of patients' presenting complaints are not investigated
- 45% of patients' presenting complaints are not elicited
- in up to 50% of consultations doctor and patient do not agree on the main presenting problem
- misunderstandings between doctors and patients seem to occur in a majority of consultations
- patients have been found to have larger and more complex agendas when consulting doctors than their doctors seem to realise
- doctors provide only limited information to patients who consistently state a preference for receiving more information from them
- doctors overestimate the time they devote to explaining things to patients
- doctors consistently use jargon patients do not understand
- patients only recall or understand a small fraction of what they are told by their doctors

A model of the encounter (Calgary–Cambridge Guides)

A range of models has been proposed to describe and guide doctors in the conduct of patient consultations. A group of teachers and researchers have endeavoured to bring together much of the research on doctor–patient communication and to provide a comprehensive model of the consultation, incorporating many elements of other models. From this work they have generated a set of guides to inform the teaching and acquisition of communication skills by healthcare professionals, known as the Calgary–Cambridge Guides – one designed for students (Silverman et al) and one for teachers (Kurtz et al – see Further Reading).

Figure 9.1 is the basic framework of the medical consultation and incorporates both clinical content and communication processes that make up the consultation. Each element

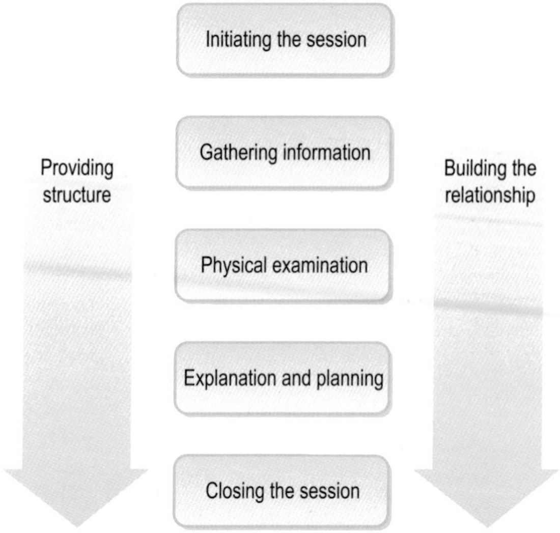

Fig. 9.1 **The enhanced Calgary–Cambridge Guide to the medical interview: the basic framework.**

of this diagram can be expanded into a more detailed set of process skills to be acquired and content to be discovered (Fig. 9.2). The full guide also contains an 'options' section under investigation and planning (see below).

Initiating the session

The key skills here involve establishing initial rapport and identifying the reasons for the consultation. Establishing initial rapport includes:

- greeting patients appropriately and getting their name
- introducing yourself, explaining your role and the nature of the interview, and obtaining consent
- demonstrating respect and interest; attending to the patient's comfort.

Identifying the reason(s) for the consultation would involve:

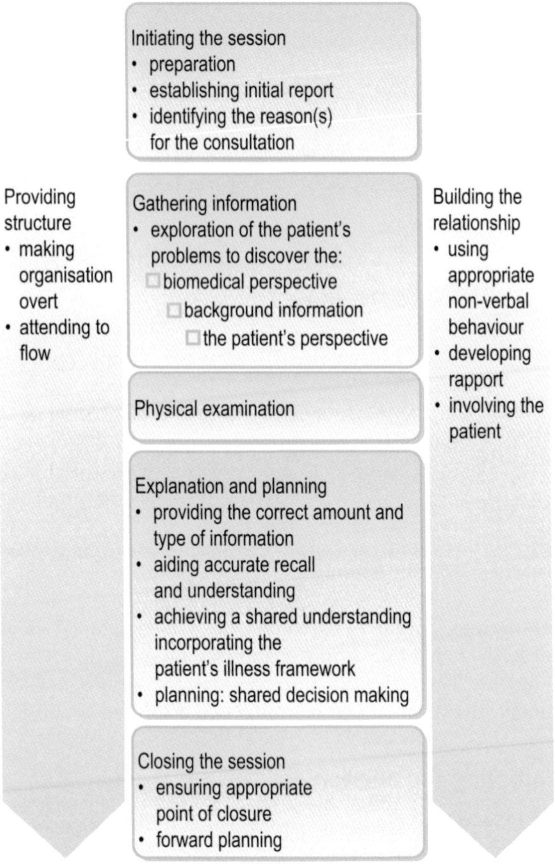

Initiating the session
- preparation
- establishing initial report
- identifying the reason(s) for the consultation

Providing structure
- making organisation overt
- attending to flow

Gathering information
- exploration of the patient's problems to discover the:
  - ☐ biomedical perspective
    - ☐ background information
      - ☐ the patient's perspective

Building the relationship
- using appropriate non-verbal behaviour
- developing rapport
- involving the patient

Physical examination

Explanation and planning
- providing the correct amount and type of information
- aiding accurate recall and understanding
- achieving a shared understanding incorporating the patient's illness framework
- planning: shared decision making

Closing the session
- ensuring appropriate point of closure
- forward planning

Fig. 9.2 **The enhanced Calgary–Cambridge Guide to the medical interview: the expanded framework.**

- identifying the patient's problems or issues using an appropriate opening question
- listening attentively to the patient's opening statement without interruption
- confirming the list of the patient's problems and screening for further problems

- negotiating the agenda to meet the needs of patient and physician.

Gathering information

The key skills here involve exploring the patient's problems and understanding the patient's perspective. Exploring the patient's problems can involve many factors:

- encouraging the patient to tell the story
- using open and closed questioning techniques appropriately
- listening attentively, avoiding interrupting the patient and allowing space for the patient to compose any thoughts
- facilitating the patient's responses verbally and non-verbally
- picking up on verbal and non-verbal cues and checking them out and acknowledging them as appropriate
- clarifying the patient's statements
- summarising periodically to verify understanding of what the patient has said
- using concise, easily understood questions and comments – avoiding or explaining jargon
- accurately establishing dates and sequences of events.

Understanding the patient's perspective will require the GP to:

- actively determine and try to appropriately explore:
  - patient's ideas
  - patient's concerns
  - patient's expectations
  - effects of problems on patient's life
- encourage the patient to express any feelings.

Providing structure to the consultation

This is a task that runs right through the consultation in parallel with the above (see Fig. 9.1). Key skills include 'making organisation overt' and 'attending to flow'. As far as making organisation overt is concerned, summarising at

271

the end of a specific line of enquiry to confirm understanding before moving on to next section will help, as will progressing from one section to another using signposting, transitional statements. Attending to flow will involve structuring the consultation in a logical sequence, attending to timing and keeping the interview on-task.

Building the relationship

There is another task that runs right through the consultation in parallel with those already mentioned (see Fig. 9.1) – building the relationship. Key skills include using appropriate non-verbal behaviour, developing rapport, and involving the patient.

Using appropriate non-verbal behaviour
- demonstrate appropriate non-verbal behaviour:
  - eye contact
  - posture, position, movement
  - vocal cues
- if reading or writing notes or using the computer, doing so in a manner that does not interfere with the dialogue or rapport
- demonstrate appropriate confidence.

Developing rapport
- accept the legitimacy of patient's views and feelings and be non-judgemental
- use empathy to communicate understanding – overtly acknowledge the patient's views and feelings
- provide support by expressing concern, understanding, willingness to help; acknowledge the patient's own coping efforts and appropriate self-care; offer partnership
- deal sensitively with embarrassing and disturbing topics and physical pain, including when associated with physical examination.

Involving the patient
- share thinking with the patient to encourage patient involvement

- explain the rationale for questions or parts of the physical examination as appropriate
- during the physical examination explain the process and seek permission as appropriate.

Explanation and planning

The key skills required in this phase of the consultation include providing the correct amount and type of information, aiding accurate recall and understanding, achieving a shared understanding incorporating the patient's perspective and planning, and sharing decision-making with the patient.

Provide the correct amount and type of information
- chunk and check, i.e. give the information in reasonable-sized chunks and check the patient understands them
- assess the patient's starting point by asking for the patient's prior knowledge early on when giving information and discover the extent of the desire for information
- ask the patient what other information would be helpful
- give explanations at appropriate times including avoiding giving advice, information or reassurance prematurely.

273

Aid accurate recall and understanding
- organise explanation by dividing into discrete sections and developing a logical sequence
- use explicit categorisation or signposting of information being given to the patient
- use repetition and summarising to reinforce information
- use concise, easily understood language and avoid or explain jargon
- use visual methods of conveying information
- check the patient's understanding.

Achieve a shared understanding incorporating the patient's perspective

- relate explanations to the patient's perspective, i.e. to previously elicited ideas, concerns and expectation
- provide opportunities and encourage the patient to contribute
- pick up and respond to verbal and non-verbal cues
- elicit patient's beliefs, reactions and feelings.

Plan, including sharing decision making with patients

- share your own thinking as appropriate
- involve the patient, e.g.:
  - offer suggestions and choices
  - encourage the patient's own ideas and suggestions
- explore management options
- ascertain the level of involvement the patient wishes in making the decision at hand
- negotiate a mutually acceptable plan
  - signpost your own position regarding available options
  - determine the patient's preferences
- check with the patient
  - if the plan is acceptable
  - if all concerns have been addressed.

Closing the session

The key skills here include forward planning and ensuring an appropriate point of closure. Forward planning includes contracting with the patient the next steps to be taken by the patient and the doctor, and providing 'safety nets' – explaining possible unexpected outcomes, what to do if the plan is not working and when and how to seek additional help. Ensuring appropriate closure will involve summarising the session briefly and clarifying the care plan, with a final check that the patient agrees with and is comfortable with the plan.

Explanation and planning in particular circumstances

In addition to these key skills, the Calgary–Cambridge Guides offer some additional guidance for special circumstances that may arise in the explanation and planning part of the consultation as detailed below. If discussing opinion and significance of problems the following skills may be required:

- offering opinion on what is going on and naming the problem if possible
- revealing the rationale for your opinion
- explaining causation, seriousness, expected outcome and short- and long-term consequences
- eliciting the patient's beliefs, reactions and concerns regarding the opinion.

If negotiating mutual plans of action the following skills may be required:

- discussing options
- providing information on action or treatment offered
- obtaining the patient's view of the need for action, perceived benefits, barriers and motivation
- accepting the patient's views advocating an alternative viewpoint if necessary
- eliciting the patient's reactions and concerns about plans and treatments, including acceptability
- taking patient's lifestyle, beliefs, cultural backgrounds and abilities into consideration
- encouraging the patient to be involved in implementing plans, to take responsibility and be self-reliant
- asking about the patient's support systems and discussing other support available.

If discussing investigations and procedures the following skills may be required:

- providing clear information on procedures
- relating procedures to the treatment plan

- encouraging questions about and discussion of potential anxieties or negative outcomes.

Demanding communication situations

While all consultations demand a high level of communication skills, there are situations in which these skills are particularly vital and must be applied with particular sensitivity and awareness of context for the communication to be successful. Examples of these situations might include:

- breaking bad news
- communicating with culturally and ethnically diverse patients
- communicating with the very young and the very old
- communicating with patients with mental health problems
- communicating over the telephone
- communicating with carers.

These situations are also covered in the books by the Calgary–Cambridge group, which spell out in detail how the guides apply in these specific situations.

Breaking bad news

It is inevitable in the practice of medicine that occasions will arise when the information we have to impart to a patient will constitute bad news. This is obviously the case when having to tell the patient they have a fatal condition but telling the patient they have a long-term condition – even one that can be treated and controlled – is also, from the patient's perspective, bad news.

It is not always possible to tell what will constitute bad news for a patient and so, while guidelines can be provided on how to impart bad news, you have to remain alert at all times to how the information you give to patients is being perceived by them. Guidelines on breaking bad news (Box 9.2) can only highlight the issues and point out pitfalls to avoid, but it is difficult to be very prescriptive on how to give any particular information to any patient, as considerable judgement has to be exercised in this delicate area.

Culturally and ethnically diverse patients

As societies become more ethnically diverse doctors are increasingly engaged in consultations with patients whose cultural and ethnic background is different from their own.

Box 9.2 Suggested guidelines for breaking bad news

- Prepare in advance of the consultation – clarify the patient's diagnosis as much as possible, what treatment can/will be offered, the range of possible prognoses with and without treatment, what the patient already knows or seems to suspect.
- Ensure the right setting for the consultation – privacy is paramount, try and ensure you will not be interrupted and have adequate time to deal with the patient's questions, make sure the patient is comfortable; try ensure that the patient has someone with them during and after the consultation.
- Find out what the patient already knows and work from there.
- Gently warn the patient bad news is coming, e.g. 'I'm afraid what I have to tell you may not be what you were hoping for'.
- Don't rush. Give the information in small amounts and watch for the patient's reaction. The patient may 'shut down' if the news is very shocking – if so, stop giving information and try and console and help the patient come to terms with any feelings.
- Repeat the information if necessary. Be prepared to repeat information several times over several consultations. Giving bad news is rarely a one-off event. Arrange to see the patient again soon.
- Be honest but not brutally so. Try to provide hope tempered with realism.
- Be prepared for your own responses, too. Giving bad news is emotionally draining and upsetting. Develop appropriate strategies for dealing with your own feelings about death, dying, etc.

Interpersonal communication is highly dependent on both parties being aware of and abiding by certain conversational rules that, while unwritten, are absorbed as part of every person's acculturation.

Fortunately some of the rules are very similar across all cultures, such as the need for two people conversing to take turns in speaking, but there are often subtle differences in the application of these rules in different cultures. However, doctors are also a distinct cultural group with their own customs (e.g. physical examination of people they meet in their work) and language (medical jargon), and so it has been argued that all doctor–patient encounters are cross-cultural events. Important points to consider about communication across a divide of language and culture are outlined in Box 9.3.

Important areas where culturally diverse groups tend to differ from the prevailing Western medicine viewpoint include:

- use of language and medical terms
- use and interpretation of body language and non-verbal communication – touch, eye contact, proximity, expression of emotion
- beliefs about the causation and treatment of illness (especially the role of diet), which overlap with morality, relationship to lifestyle and life events and expectations of 'cure'
- attitudes to sex, sexuality, fertility and fertility control, childbirth
- attitudes to death and dying, to loss, to bereavement, to bad news
- attitudes to use/misuse of drugs including tobacco and alcohol
- attitudes and typical responses to ethical issues.

Communicating with the elderly

With the improving health of the population the proportion of elderly is increasing – for most doctors communicating with elderly patients is a more and more frequent occurrence. While the skills required are the same as for

Box 9.3 Communicating across a divide of language and culture

- Culture has a major bearing on how patients communicate and on their perceptions and beliefs about health and illness. These need to be taken into consideration in the medical encounter.
- Virtually all patients are culturally different and use language differently from their doctor. Be alert to these differences. Assume as little as possible and check your assumptions about what patients mean by what they say – and what they understand of what you say – as often as possible.
- With patients who are obviously from a different cultural background try and learn as much as possible about their attitudes to illness, their beliefs about the causes and manifestations of their health problem(s), and what their expectations of care are, before deciding on treatment of their problem(s). If you have a practice in which one particular ethnic or cultural minority predominates, time spent learning about the details of that culture will be rewarded in more fruitful medical encounters.
- Beware of assuming that, because patients come from a particular cultural background, they share all of the beliefs, customs and attitudes of that group. Knowledge of these, while useful, is only a guide. Check with patients individually about where they stand on important issues in their medical care.
- With patients who speak a different language it is important to use interpreters or interpretation services to understand as much as possible about their problem(s) and their own views of their problem(s). Interpreters should, ideally, be trained in interpretation in the medical context. They should be trained to convey accurately all of what the patient says (rather than placing their own interpretation on what the patient means) and be able to convey contextual insights on verbal and non-verbal communication in their linguistico-cultural group. Family members are not ideal interpreters but are often the only option available. They should be told to repeat exactly what the patient says (rather than interpreting it themselves). If the doctor is worried that the family

Box 9.3 *Continued*.

   member might be harming or controlling the patient, it
may be necessary to arrange to see the patient again with
an independent interpreter.
- Where a doctor practices with many patients from a
particular language group it is worthwhile learning some of
that language – basic medical terminology at least.

other patients, elderly patients may present particular
challenges.

   Firstly, they may have different perspectives on health
and illness from younger patients, but not always what you
might expect. Elderly patients, even of the same age, vary
dramatically in their attitudes to the possibility of dying
from their illness. Secondly, loss of physical or mental
faculties can make communication more difficult and less
reliable. Finally, be alert to the possibility of ageism in your
own thinking. Studies have shown that doctors often have
a certain nihilism in their therapeutic decision-making
based on a patient's age – sometimes denying or less actively
pursuing treatment in older patients, even when the elderly
patient might benefit as much as, or possibly even more so,
than a younger patient (Box 9.4).

Communicating with children and parents

Consultations with children are particularly challenging in
several respects. Firstly, most consultations with children
will take place in the presence of a parent or guardian – the
addition of further participants to a consultation inevitably
complicates matters and requires the doctor to be aware
of several dynamics simultaneously (see multi-person
consultations, below). Secondly, children vary greatly in
their ability to describe their symptoms and in their understanding of illness and health matters. These capabilities
vary not only with age but also from child to child, even
within the same age group. Thirdly, consultations with children and their parents are very often imbued with anxiety
– sometimes on the part of the child, sometimes on the part
of the parent and sometimes both. Furthermore, both child

Box 9.4 **Key points in communicating with the elderly**

- Be prepared to listen and take time. For patients with hearing or speech difficulties extra time and skill will be needed and this should be scheduled for, to avoid communication being neglected.
- Older patients often have longer and more complex medical histories. A judgement has to be made about how much detail is required and skill and sensitivity is needed in guiding the patient to give the information deemed useful and relevant and avoiding excessive detail that might be less important.
- Don't make assumptions about what the older patient might want by way of investigations or treatment. Check with them.
- Be careful not to get involved in communications with and making decisions with relatives or carers without involving the older person. It is generally preferable that communication about the illness, its prognosis and management be conducted with the patient and carers or relatives together.
- Try to ageism-proof your behaviour and decisions about older patients. Ask yourself recurrently if you are reacting or behaving differently or coming to different decisions based on age – would you be doing anything differently for a younger patient?

and parent may have difficulties in either recognising or expressing their anxieties (Box 9.5).

Communicating with the mentally ill

The presence of a mental illness can interfere with communication in a variety of ways. Depressed patients may be reluctant to engage in dialogue. A psychotic patient may struggle to converse in an understandable fashion. As a consequence of the prevalence of such difficulties in mental ill health a collateral history from another witness is often an essential element in putting together the full picture to arrive at an accurate diagnosis.

Box 9.5 Some suggestions for communicating with children and parents

- Always try to engage in some communication with the child patient. Do not interact exclusively with the parent(s) or guardian.
- With very small children eye contact and reassuring words may be sufficient.
- The older the child the more you can reasonably engage them in the consultations. Children from school age onwards will be more used to talking with non-familiar adults and can be invited to give their own account of their problem.
- Adolescents generally appreciate an opportunity to converse with the doctor on their own and, if they are assured of confidentiality and feel they can trust the doctor, they may disclose important information one-to-one that they will not divulge in the presence of a parent or guardian. Strictly speaking, parental permission is required to consult with children under 16 on their own.
- An awareness of the linguistic and cognitive developmental milestones of children and the ages at which they are typically achieved is helpful to tailoring communication with children.
- Most children are happier to be addressed by their first names. Use simple language appropriate to the child's age but beware of being patronising.
- Seek the views of the children and the relevant adults on the problem and its suggested solution(s).
- Children with continuing medical needs should be actively involved in the care of their own illness in an age-appropriate manner. For example, children with asthma should be encouraged to take some responsibility for the self-administration of their inhalers.
- Look out for cues, particularly regarding the relationship between the child and any accompanying adult. The presence of both parents is often an expression of a higher than average level of anxiety about the child's problem. It can also, however, occasionally be indicative of parental disharmony or mistrust or, more benignly, a sign of more than usually equal maternal and paternal involvement in direct care of the child, or sometimes is just a matter of convenience.

Communicating with depressed patients

Building rapport is vital to establishing the relationship with depressed patients so that they will 'open up' to the doctor and disclose how they are actually feeling. It may be more useful, initially, to get patients to describe their feelings and to try and empathise with them before trying to get an historical account of the development of the illness or exploring the actual symptom pattern. Patients are often reluctant to admit to symptoms of depression because of the stigma that attaches to mental illness – they may require reassurance that their doctor does not hold any such stigmatic view of them or their illness. Suicidal ideation must always be explored in depressed patients (see Chapter 3) but this must be done with great sensitivity and a good deal of self-confidence to display that the doctor is neither shocked nor judging the patient for having suicidal thoughts or intentions.

Communicating with psychotic patients

Psychosis is characterised by thought disorder, hallucinations and delusions and is compounded, very often, by a lack of insight. These obviously impede ordinary dialogue as they can produce strange and difficult to understand responses to the questions a doctor might ask, as well as misunderstanding of who or what the doctor is. Furthermore, psychotic patients are generally anxious, may be paranoid and may even be inclined to violence.

283

First try and find out as much as possible from third parties about how the patient has presented. Is there any past history? Has the patient expressed paranoid ideas or been violent? A psychotic patient will often feel mistrustful and misunderstood by others and so initial effort needs to be put into trying to gain the patient's trust. Giving the impression of understanding what is going on for the patient, while not actually colluding with their mistaken beliefs or false perceptions, is the ideal balance. While negotiating a treatment plan may be the ideal, this may be a situation where reaching an acceptable compromise with the patient may not be possible and compulsory admission may, ultimately, be required.

Communicating over the telephone

Communication with patients over the telephone is increasingly popular with both patients and doctors. Patients may value the more ready access to medical advice and being saved all the trouble and possible delay involved in getting a face-to-face consultation. Where the patient pays directly for a consultation (e.g. for a large proportion of the population in the Republic of Ireland, see Chapter 11) a telephone consultation may well be free or is, at least, likely to be cheaper.

Doctors may also value telephone consultations, particularly if they can obviate the need for a home visit or an out-of-hours call. However, there are substantial disadvantages to doctors, who may be expected to reach a diagnosis and/or agree a management plan without the benefits of seeing the patient and in the absence of the usual non-verbal communication. These problems are compounded by the inability to observe the patient's general condition and to assess any clinical signs.

To compensate for the lack of non-verbal communication, you must pay extra attention to all aspects of verbal communication, including indications from the quality of the voice of how the patient is feeling, e.g. angry, depressed or anxious. You need to listen very carefully to what is said and keep checking with the patient that your understanding of what has been said squares with theirs. To replace the usual non-verbal signals you may need to use more facilitative utterances (such as 'umm', 'go on', 'tell me more' etc.) to encourage the patient to continue talking.

You are also totally dependent on the history to reach a diagnosis, or at least rule out any significant risk of a serious health problem, so the history must be taken with extra care. You need to be particularly sensitive to all cues and respond to them clearly and verbally. The use of leading or closed questions can be particularly misleading when not in the presence of the patient. Due to the additional hazards in telephone consulting it is imperative that the patient is clearly instructed to make further contact if symptoms persist or worsen or if new symptoms develop. This is a form of 'safety netting' (see Chapter 2).

Multi-person consultations

General practice consultations usually tend to involve only one person and the doctor. However, there are circumstances in which more than one person attends and is involved in the consultation. These place additional demands on doctors and their communication skills. Common examples of multi-person consultations include:

- consultations attended by a child or children accompanied by a parent or parents (see above)
- consultations by both parties to a stable emotional relationship (mostly heterosexual couples but can be homosexual couples too)
- consultations with patients (typically elderly patients) accompanied by carers (who can be relatives or other informal carers or occasionally formal carers such as social workers).

With the exception of consultations with babies, one of the principal requirements is to address both parties, i.e. try not to ignore one party simply because another tends to dominate the interaction. In multi-person situations it is sometimes desirable to ask one party to leave the consultation to get another to speak freely and to get both sides of the story. Seeing parties separately may be particularly necessary if some discord between them becomes apparent.

Reasons people have for attending together include:

- simple practical convenience
- in order to lend moral support to an ill person and perhaps even help them challenge the doctor
- to ensure that the patient 'tells the doctor everything' or that everything the doctor tells the patient is known by the carers.

It is important to recognise when the attendance of more than one person is purely a practical matter, e.g. it was more convenient to attend together, or whether the joint attendance has significance beyond that – to miss this significance can lead to an inappropriate response by the doctor.

Communicating with carers and relatives

Although it is generally preferable to communicate with relatives and carers in the presence of the patient, this is not always possible. Explicit consent must be obtained from the patient, wherever possible, to discussions with carers taking place in the absence of the patient. In obtaining such consent you should try to specify what is going to be discussed with the relative or carer, although you cannot always allow for issues that might arise unexpectedly during a consultation.

Avoid saying things about patients that you would not be happy to say to them face-to-face. More often, though, it is the relatives or carers who have information for the GP that they would, perhaps, not be happy to say to the patient face-to-face. While you can generally rely on the testimony of relatives and carers and on the bona fides of their concern, you must be alert to the possibility that relatives and carers can have more ulterior motives in giving certain information to a doctor.

Your primary loyalty should always be to the patient. When it comes to talking to relatives the general skills and attitudes required for communication with patients apply to this form of consultation, too. Thus, even when you have information you want to impart to the relatives or carers you should start by listening to what they have to say and to understand the knowledge base from which the relative or carer is coming.

The doctor–patient relationship

Successive consultations between a doctor and patient build into a relationship. The nature of this relationship contributes greatly to the effectiveness of the doctor and, hence, the quality of care experienced by the patient. Stewart and Roter

Table 9.1
Different types of doctor–patient relationship (after Stewart & Roter 1989)

	Patient passive	Patient active
Doctor active	Paternalistic	Mutualistic
Doctor passive	Laissez faire	Consumerist

have described four main types of doctor–patient relationship (Table 9.1):

- *the traditional 'paternalistic' relationship*, in which the doctor is in charge and the patient passively accepts the doctor's complete authority
- *the consumerist relationship*, in which the patient has a much greater say to the extent of dictating the acceptable type or extent of care to the doctor
- *the laissez-faire relationship*, in which the doctor leaves decisions to the patient but the patient does not take up the responsibility, and in which neither doctor nor patient are effectively in charge
- *the mutualistic relationship*, in which doctor and patient are actively involved and both contribute to decision-making on an equal basis.

In their model, mutualistic doctor–patient relationships are taken to develop from the application of 'patient-centred medicine' to successive consultations. Patient centredness is a philosophy of medical practice and not just a technique for the conduct of consultations. It is an approach to doctor–patient relationships where the doctor seeks to work more closely in an equal partnership with patients in caring for their health and managing their illnesses. It is particularly appropriate in an era when the relationship between professionals and their clients is changing generally towards one of greater egalitarianism. Patients are also better informed and have a much larger role in managing their own ill health, especially so in the case of chronic ill health.

Relationships in hospital and general practice

While relationships between doctors and patients are broadly similar in all clinical settings, relationships can develop in general practice in ways that are appreciably different from those usually developed in hospital settings. These differences are summarised in Table 9.2. The type of relationship generally possible in general practice has certain advantages. It provides more scope for the exploration of psychosocial issues:

- diagnosis may be facilitated by the greater knowledge the GP will typically have of the patient's medical and psychosocial background
- it facilitates the GP's use of a sort of 'sixth sense' whereby flashes of inspiration seem to occur that may cut to the chase
- the patient will usually be more at ease and may find it easier to express underlying worries or other underlying agendas
- reassurance may be more effective both because the GP may have a better feeling for what is worrying the patient and because the reassurance given is more trusted

Table 9.2
Contrasts between hospital and GP doctor–patient relationships

General practice	Hospital
Initiated by patient	Contact initiated by GP (not usually by the patient)
Encounters brief (5–10 mins) but may be very numerous	Encounter length varies (can be long) but not that many encounters in total
Intervals between consultations may be short	Intervals between encounters either very short (daily or more frequent, inpatients) or very long (typically outpatients)
Relationship expected to be long-term	Relationship is one-off or episodic
More social content	Less social content
More intimate	More formal
Mutuality easier to achieve	Paternalism more typical

- trust in the familiar doctor can also facilitate adherence to the treatment regimen prescribed (see also Chapter 7).

Further Reading

Freeling P, Harris C M 1984 The doctor–patient relationship, 3rd edn. Churchill Livingstone, Edinburgh

Kurtz S, Silverman J, Draper J 2005 Teaching and learning communication skills in medicine, 2nd edn. Radcliffe Medical Press, Oxford (designed for teachers)

Lloyd M, Bor R 1996 Communications skills for medicine. Churchill Livingstone, Edinburgh

Neighbour R 2004 The inner consultation: how to develop an effective and intuitive consulting style, 2nd edn. Radcliffe Medical Press, Oxford

Silverman J, Kurtz S, Draper J 2005 Skills for communicating with patients, 2nd edn. Radcliffe Medical Press, Oxford (designed for students)

Stewart M, Roter D 1989 Communicating with medical patients. Sage Publications, London

Stewart M, Brown J, Weston W, McWhinney I, McWilliam C, Freeman T 2003 Patient-centred medicine: transforming the clinical method, 2nd edn. Radcliffe Medical Press, Oxford

The primary care team

Traditionally GPs worked on their own, sometimes from their own homes. However, as general practice has developed, they have begun to work with other doctors in group practices, supported by other staff, from premises specifically for the purpose of the delivery of primary healthcare. This development pattern is mirrored throughout most of the developed world, although progressing at different rates in different healthcare systems. Primary healthcare physicians and the other people with whom they work are referred to as the 'primary healthcare team'.

The composition of the primary care team varies from time to time and from place to place. Two distinct types of team can be identified. 'Functional teams' consist of the individuals involved in the delivery of care to specific patients. The 'structural team' is more of a virtual team which consists of all the various people and agencies that are extant and, at least potentially, available to assist in the provision of care to individuals or populations.

The functional team

The most basic functional team that is commonly seen in general practice comprises the GP, a nurse (who may be a practice nurse or a district nurse) and a receptionist or other administrative person. Depending on the nature of the patient's problem and the availability of staff, this functional team may sometimes be larger. For example, in the case of a patient receiving palliative care the functional team may comprise the doctor, a palliative home care nurse or MacMillan nurse, a district nurse, a palliative care doctor, administrative staff of both the practice and the hospice and, possibly, a lay volunteer from the hospice.

The functional team need not even involve the doctor. Many women and their babies in the post-partum period are looked after by a midwife and a health visitor with little or no involvement of the doctor. Lay carers can also be considered to be part of the functional team as they are effectively co-workers in the provision of care (indeed, they are often providing the bulk of the care). As team members they ought to be kept in the communication loop when the next steps in care are being considered. The functional team is focused on the function of providing care.

The structural team

The structural team can be very large indeed. Box 10.1 lists the various health professionals who might be part of the team. To this list can be added various administrative staff in the practice (secretaries, receptionists, practice managers) and in various community care agencies. One can also include the clergy and various non-statutory agencies, which may be generic (such as care of the elderly) or disease-specific (such as Diabetes UK and the Diabetes Federation in Ireland). Finally, there are all the members of the local

Box 10.1   Potential members of the structural primary care team

- GPs
- District nurse
- Practice nurse
- Health visitor
- Midwife
- Physiotherapist
- Occupational therapist
- Pharmacist
- Dentist
- Speech and language therapist
- Audiologist
- Psychologist
- Social worker
- Counsellor
- Community paediatrician
- Community geriatrician
- Specialist/outreach nurses
- Nursing/rest home staff
- Patient participation group

community who, at least potentially, may slot into the role of carer if circumstance demands it. The involvement of various members will, obviously, vary greatly from case to case.

This broad concept of the structural team is useful as it serves as a reminder of the very wide range of options that may be available to a doctor or functional team in looking after a patient. It is also useful to consider various subsets of this group when thinking strategically about the future development of the practice as they may be useful people to consult or even involve in the planning process.

The nature of primary care teams

Primary care teams are particularly characterised by:

- flexible leadership
- blurred interprofessional boundaries.

Flexible leadership

In Chapter 1 it was noted that primary care teams differ from hospital teams in being non-hierarchical and more egalitarian. This does not mean, however, that they are leaderless but rather that the leadership is not fixed – it can move around the group according to the needs of the patient. Thus for a patient with a predominantly medical problem, such as an acute infection, the team leader may be the doctor. For a patient with primarily nursing needs, such as a patient convalescing from surgery, the nurse may assume a leadership role. For those with a particular problem demanding certain skills another team member may assume the leadership role – an example might be the physiotherapist in respect of a post-stroke patient.

Doctors still have a large share of the leadership, particularly in respect of the overall running of the practice and in the setting and maintaining of clinical standard, as they carry a large part of the burden of medico-legal responsibility. Increasingly, professionalised practice managers are also developing a major strategic leadership role. Responsibilities for clinical standards, traditionally the responsibility of the individual GP, are coming to be shared with primary care groups.

Blurred inter-professional boundaries

As well as flexible leadership, primary care teams usually have weaker and less distinct inter-professional boundaries than would be found in hospitals. Thus doctors may, for instance, take bloods and do dressings, tasks that in hospitals are done by phlebotomists and nurses. Likewise, nurses and other team members may take on tasks traditionally associated with doctors such as making diagnoses and recommending treatment. This flexibility is driven by the nature of general practice, which is focused on the needs of patients rather than the professional boundaries of service providers. General practice functions more effectively on the basis of relationships rather than of roles. Thus, particularly in situations in which counselling or listening and talking are a large part of the therapeutic response, it may matter more to the patient who is dealing with them more than what their specific professional qualifications or roles are.

The task of breaking bad news to a patient is an example. While this might be seen as the role of the doctor, the patient may ask their questions and hope for answers from any member of the primary care team, including administrative staff. While it is important for people not to stray too far from their areas of competence, it should be within their capacity to respond, at least in a limited way, and to try and deal with the issue or issues patients raise with them. The scope for other team members to respond to the needs presented to them can be greatly enhanced by training and by the development of protocols for dealing with situations that might otherwise lie outside people's basic competences.

Teamworking

For functional teams to work successfully there are certain prerequisites. These include:

- shared goals
- mutual respect
- good communication
- mutual understanding and respect for each other's contribution to the team effort
- a great deal of flexibility
- a good understanding of each other's abilities and capacities and each other's limitations
- a shared commitment to an egalitarian style of working.

These requirements are best met if each team member knows something of the background and training of their fellow workers. Teamworking is also facilitated by regular meetings at which the tasks in hand are shared and where more general and strategic issues, such as shared goals, can also be raised. Communication can be facilitated by shared care cards or records on which all team members can record their findings, conclusions and treatment plans for the patient. Training in teamworking also helps – the seeds for this can be sewn in basic training by different professions sharing educational experiences.

Barriers to good teamworking include:

- poor communication or mis-communication
- lack of understanding of each other's roles
- too fixed ideas of what other team members can and should do
- differentials in pay and status and being employed within different management structures answerable to different authorities
- lack of clarity about leadership (while leadership should be flexible it must also be clear at all times who actually is in charge).

Non-hierarchical working implies that efforts are made to move forward on the basis of consensus wherever possible and appropriate. However, decisions often have to be made within specific, and usually quite short, timescales. This can thwart efforts at consensus building. Therefore, there needs to be clarity about who can make what decisions in the absence of a consensus. This often falls to doctors because the burden of medico-legal responsibility belongs largely to them.

GPs occasionally have to draw on the services of people and agencies from beyond the close functional team. Working with people you don't know so well requires a different approach, although the general principles of team working still apply. Thus, for example, when working with voluntary groups you should have a reasonable understanding of the philosophy and background of the group. You should also understand that people in voluntary groups may not all be paid for what they do and so you cannot so easily make specific or elaborate demands of them.

When working with other social agencies – for example social welfare agencies – you should appreciate that such agencies are governed by regulations and resource constraints that may restrict what they can do in response to your requests for assistance on behalf of a patient. You must also try to comply with whatever bureaucratic procedures are needed to allow benefit agencies to activate their assistance mechanisms.

Doctors work with a great variety of agencies, many spanning the boundaries between medicine and other aspects of society. The Coroner is one such example who straddles some of the boundaries between the practice of medicine and the requirements of the law. The Coroner has specific roles – such as in the investigation of suspicious deaths – that mean doctors are obliged to cooperate in certain ways with that function. There is legislation governing such matters and doctors should be familiar with it. These matters are described in texts and courses on forensic medicine but are touched on here to remind readers that Coroners (and, indeed, other agencies of law enforcement such as the police) should also be regarded as members of the healthcare team – albeit with a somewhat different agenda. Similar principles apply to ensuring that this aspect of teamworking is also successful.

Background, training and roles of members

General practitioner

Background and training

General practitioners are medically qualified doctors who have taken a period of additional training specifically for general practice. This additional training is specified by a European Union directive and currently consists of two years of hospital training in specialties regarded as relevant to general practice (such as internal medicine, geriatrics, paediatrics, psychiatry etc.) and a further year of training in a designated training general practice – all taken after completion of the pre-registration house officer year.

During the general practice training year doctors in training will also attend a 'day release' programme, during which the philosophy and practice of general practice is studied in more depth. In some regions all three years of postgraduate training required for general practice can be obtained as a 'package' and full-day or half-day release may also be undertaken during the two hospital years. On successful completion of training doctors are issued with a Certificate of Satisfactory Completion of Training, which is a prerequisite for obtaining a job as GP in the UK. Broadly similar provisions regarding GP training apply in the Republic of Ireland, except that it now comprises two years of hospital training followed by two years of training in general practice or in the community.

Functions

The doctor's functions are the diagnosis, management, and prevention of disease. In all of these functions, though, the GP is assisted by other members of the team. Increasingly, the doctor's role is changing to one of overseeing and directing the work of others in respect of routine problems and cases, as well as dealing with those cases where diagnosis or management is more challenging. GPs carry primary responsibility for the care of patients – they, arguably, have the heaviest burden of responsibility if things go wrong – and so it is important that they delegate work effectively to other team members and monitor their activities to ensure care is being delivered to the required standards.

GPs also play an important role in the lives of patients that goes beyond mere technical care of their problems. It has more to do with 'being there' for patients when required, being committed and trustworthy. This function is also sometimes shared with other team members but it is not one that can be delegated. Patients decide in whom they invest trust and expect to 'be there' for them.

Nurses

Box 10.2 lists the different kinds of nurse active in primary care.

Background and training

In their basic education all nurses learn anatomy, physiology, pathology, pharmacology, medicine, and surgery –

Box 10.2 **Different kinds of primary care nurse**

- Practice nurses
- District nurses
- Health visitors
- Community midwives
- Community psychiatric nurses
- Clinical nurse specialists
- Nurse practitioners

though possibly not in the same depth as medical students. Nursing courses vary with regard to whether they offer paediatrics, obstetrics, psychiatry, public health and community nursing as part of basic education – although all these are options available as postgraduate courses. They are also taught behavioural sciences (psychology, sociology etc.) and may have had more exposure to these subjects than doctors, although medical curricula are now also embracing these subjects for medical graduates too.

Other major components of basic nurse training consist of clinical placements. Nurses have highly developed skills in forming close nurturing and more power-balanced relationships with patients than doctors. Nurses follow protocols and guidelines more diligently than doctors. Protocols have, traditionally, been a more significant component of nurse training.

Functions

Practice nurses are registered nurses who can have a wide variety of different experience before coming into practice nursing. Increasingly, practice nurses will have undertaken specific courses in practice nursing but these are not yet a prerequisite for a career in practice nursing. Practice nurses are generally appointed at the discretion of individual GPs or practices. They undertake a very diverse range of activities from the traditional nursing roles of doing dressings, taking bloods, cervical cytology smears and carrying out ECGs, to more active roles in health promotion, chronic disease management and management of minor and self-limiting illnesses.

Practice nurses differ from other primary care nurses in that they are employed by the GP or GPs in a practice rather than by a health authority or equivalent. The types of care they provide and the standards they work to are usually governed by protocols or directives from their employers. Under provisions of recent health reforms in the UK an increasing proportion of practice nurses are allowed to prescribe for patients.

District nurses

District nurses have first to qualify as state registered nurses and then acquire additional qualifications in community nursing and midwifery. They have a wide range of functions, though the bulk of their work is usually concerned with the care of the elderly. Patients are mostly referred to them on discharge from hospital or by GPs, although they may be referred by a wide variety of agencies. They usually begin their contact with a patient with a detailed assessment of the patient's nursing needs. On the basis of this they will usually then devise a care plan which they alone, or in conjunction with others (including the patient's GP), will strive to deliver. They will dress patient's wounds, help with care of stomata, and assist with bathing and general care of patients in the home environment – as well as training others (including patients and carers) in these tasks.

They also have an important role in the promotion of clients' health. Their roles may sometimes overlap with those of practice nurses, midwives, health visitors and various clinical nurse specialists, but in better functioning teams these professional nurses will divide roles and tasks between them – ideally on the basis of dialogue and agreements concerning the patients' needs and how best to meet them.

Health visitors

Health visitors are also state registered nurses who have taken additional qualifications in health visiting. Many will have had community experience prior to training as health visitors and some also have qualifications in paediatric nursing and midwifery. Their role is focused primarily on children, in respect of whom they have some statutory obligations with regard to assessment during the first year of life. As well as making regular assessments of children's development and supporting parents in their child-rearing role, especially in early life, they perform a general monitoring role and may work in liaison with others, such as GPs and social workers, in the prevention of child abuse. Where children are identified as being at risk of abuse or neglect, they will have a crucial role in subsequent care, monitoring and child protection. For children in general they are key professionals in the maintenance and promotion of health – taking over this role from the midwife at 21 days after birth and transferring responsibility to the school nursing service when the child enters the education system (usually at age 4 to 5).

Community midwives

Community midwives are also registered nurses with additional training and qualifications in midwifery. They provide various levels of service to expectant mothers and their newborn children – depending on the wishes of the mother and the type of obstetric care agreed between her, her GP and obstetrician (if any). Thus community midwives will provide home delivery for mothers for whom this is the agreed plan, provide domiciliary in and out delivery (DOMINO – which includes intra-partum care) when this is the agreed option, and routine antenatal and postnatal care for women receiving the usual standard obstetric shared care. They will usually operate antenatal clinics in conjunction with appropriately trained and registered GPs on the obstetric list and provide postnatal care to mother and baby, usually visiting them frequently at home in the early days following delivery.

Community psychiatric nurses

Community psychiatric nurses are registered nurses with specific qualifications in care of the mentally ill. They will usually work as part of a mental health care team, often under the direction of a liaison psychiatrist. They offer a variety of modes of mental health care to psychiatric patients living in the community, including monitoring and support to the long-term mentally ill, counselling or psychotherapy, and administration of depot medicine and/or supervised administration of oral medicines in some instances. They may be able to assist in the management of cases of acute mental breakdown either by collaboration with GPs and/or social workers, including voluntary or involuntary admission to hospital, or, where systems are appropriately set up, in providing community-based crisis management (see Chapter 8).

Clinical nurse specialists

There are an increasingly wide variety of nurses who provide care and support for patients suffering from a variety of illnesses. Examples include diabetes nurse specialists, continence nurses, stoma nurses, respiratory care nurses, palliative care nurses and so on. In general, such nurses come from secondary care and remain integral members of the secondary care team but they come to minister to patients in the primary care setting. They may function in one of two ways, or sometimes in a mixture of both. They can take over the patient's care from the existing nurses and doctors or, increasingly commonly, they leave the existing primary care team as the principal carers and operate more in the background – guiding existing functional primary care teams.

Nurse practitioner/advanced nurse practitioner

Nurse practitioners are nurses who perform some of the diagnostic and treatment roles traditionally performed by doctors, often in addition to more traditional nursing roles.

They are particularly active in the diagnosis and management of acute self-limiting illnesses and in chronic disease management. In the latter they undertake a more active role in patient assessment and clinical management decision-making than would be traditional for nurses. They operate to protocols agreed with medical colleagues but they usually have more latitude to make their own clinical judgements than other primary care nurses. They have additional training in diagnosis and management and may be active prescribers of drugs – often from a wider range than other nurses.

Practice receptionist/secretary

The role of the practice receptionist is a difficult and demanding one, given that it is often the first point of contact between the patient, who may be in some distress, and the practice. The holders of these positions are required to have very special qualities including:

- high level communication skills
- great tolerance – sometimes in the face of anger and abuse
- an ability to juggle many pressing demands from both patients and healthcare professionals.

In spite of these fairly arduous demands there are no specific qualifications required to become a practice receptionist. They may be appointed by GPs or practices on the basis of their best judgement. However, there are an increasing number who have either generic or specific receptionist training and/or qualifications, though many seem to acquire most of their skills 'on the job'. Many will have generic secretarial skills or qualifications, in addition, and in many practices the roles of secretary and receptionist may be combined, with some staff fulfilling each of the roles for part of their time. As well as receiving patients at the front desk and answering patient requests and queries per phone, receptionists and secretaries will fulfil a large number of other administrative duties such as filing patient records, operating call and recall systems, repeat prescribing systems and so on.

Practice manager

Nearly all practices, even quite small ones, have a practice manager – or at least a senior receptionist who fulfils this function. The practice manager is responsible for both day-to-day and, increasingly, strategic management of the practice – supported in this role by either the GPs as a group or possibly by a senior or administrative partner in the practice. The manager looks after all the administrative functions of the practice including the smooth running of the information and records systems, appointment systems (where applicable), systems for dealing with other issues (such as repeat prescribing and call and recall of patients for preventive medicine activities), financial aspects of the practice and personnel issues.

The manager will also have a major role in the practice's dealings with external agencies such as the Primary Care Trust (see Chapter 11) and in meeting various reporting and accountability responsibilities such as the production of annual reports, drug budgeting etc. The manager is also usually the person charged with the setting up and functioning of a practice's internal complaints procedures. It is a very diverse and demanding role. Practice managers may have generic management qualifications and experience but increasingly they can acquire specific qualifications in practice management from bodies such as AMSPAR (the Association of Medical Secretaries, Practice Managers, Administrators and Receptionists).

Physiotherapist

Some practices, especially larger ones, will have a physiotherapist. They have specific qualifications in physiotherapy and usually some additional post-qualification experience in hospital physiotherapy before becoming a community physiotherapist. They offer a broad range of services similar to those offered by hospital physiotherapists but with more emphasis, perhaps, on the wider range of minor musculoskeletal problems seen in general practice and on sports injuries. They can offer a range of manipulation therapies, radiation and faradic stimulation therapies, in addition to specific exercises and patient education for the self-

management of patients' conditions. Their roles can sometimes overlap with those of occupational therapists with
whom they should, ideally, work in close liaison.

Counsellor

Many practices now either employ or have access to the
services of one or more counsellors. They may be dedicated
to specific areas of counselling (such as relationship or
bereavement) or they may offer generic services for a very
wide range of psychological and social problems. More specialist counsellors may be available through agencies dedicated to a certain sphere of activity such as Relate (which
specialises in relationships). Counsellors hold a wide variety
of qualifications but the better qualified will usually hold a
degree in psychology or social work and additional qualifications in counselling and/or clinical psychology.

They have in common an approach to problems that is
focused on helping patients provide their own solutions.
They will, typically, adopt a non-judgemental approach,
seek to get the patients or clients to clarify the problem, and
then assist them in finding feasible solutions to that problem
or difficulty. Finally, they will support them in their endeavours to implement their chosen solution or solutions. They
are most helpful, therefore, where a patient has a problem
that is largely social or psychological, where they are likely
to be able to generate appropriate solutions or resolutions to
their own difficulties.

Social worker

Social workers are employed by social services agencies or
by voluntary bodies. They will often be specialised to some
extent in one or other of the following areas of practice:

- child welfare and protection
- mental health care
- care of the elderly.

They have certain statutory responsibilities – particularly
with regard to child protection, where they will be con-
strained by the legislation to act in particular ways regarding children at risk. For instance, they will have to act on

any suspicions raised to them, say by a doctor, and report suspected child abuse to the police. They are also involved in assessment and placement of children for fostering and adoption. They also work in support of families in difficulty, often working in or along with family support centres.

With regard to the mentally ill, they have a legally speci-fied role in the compulsory admission procedures and have a major role in the assessment and support of the long-term mentally ill in the community. Ideally, they should work in close liaison with community psychiatric nurses, commu-nity/liaison psychiatrists, and GPs. In relation to the elderly, they also have an assessment and placement role, as well as assisting in the provision of community and financial support.

Social workers are often perceived as the route to access-ing benefits and other social welfare provision. Social workers do, indeed, have a major role in ensuring that people access benefits but this is not their sole or main role. Helping people access the benefits system is strictly speak-ing the role of Community Welfare Officers and non-statutory bodies such as the Citizens Advice Bureau. Social workers will usually have a primary degree in either social sciences or psychology and postgraduate qualifications in social work itself.

Community pharmacist

Community pharmacists work mostly in retail pharmacies. A proportion of pharmacists are owners of their own premises and are, effectively, individual small entrepre-neurs. However, a large number of pharmacies are now owned by firms such as Boots and Lloyds, who employ pharmacists within their stores. The key legal role per-formed by pharmacists is to be responsible for the dispens-ing of medicines – specifically those medicines designated prescription-only (see Chapter 7). They also have an impor-tant role in advising all customers on the safe and effective use of medicines, in particular those medicines that are only available in pharmacies, i.e. pharmacy-only and prescription-only medicines.

Many pharmacists are seeking to widen their role in the healthcare system. Some provide preventive medicine procedures such as blood pressure measurement and choles-terol testing. Others provide pharmacy support to elderly persons' homes, nursing homes and other long-stay institu-tions. Some provide support and advice on medicines use and on the implementation of drug budgets in practices or at Primary Care Trust level (see Chapter 11). Others may provide more ad hoc drug information services.

Pharmacists qualify by taking an approved undergradu-ate degree course followed by a pre-registration year, which may be in community or hospital pharmacy. They may then register as Members of the Royal Pharmaceutical Society of Great Britain (RPSGB). In their undergraduate course they learn a certain amount of general medicine and about the diagnosis and treatment of disease but their main expertise is on all aspects of drugs, where their knowledge base will generally exceed that of the average GP.

The new GMS contract

In April 2004 a new contract for General Medical Services was implemented in the UK. A key departure in the new contract is that it is an agreement between Primary Care Organisations (PCOs) and practices rather than a contract with individual GPs. Thus the delivery on the contract is now a team responsibility. Another notable feature of the new contract is the Quality and Outcomes Framework, which provides financial incentives for practices to provide care to specified standards in a range of areas (see Chapter 5 for some of the standards relating to chronic diseases). Many of these standards, particularly those relating to prac-tice organisation, are unlikely to be achieved by doctors alone and will require a team effort (Box 10.3).

Teams in the Republic of Ireland

Primary healthcare teams are generally less well developed in Ireland than they are in the UK. General practices tend to be smaller and, while most now will employ secretaries/

Box 10.3 Domains of the quality and outcomes framework – new GMS contract

(i) clinical standards, covering coronary heart disease (CHD), stroke or transient ischaemic attacks, hypertension, diabetes, chronic obstructive pulmonary disease (COPD), epilepsy, cancer, mental health, hypothyroidism and asthma

(ii) organisational standards, covering records and information about patients, information for patients, education and training, practice management and medicines management

(iii) experience of patients, covering the services provided, how they are provided and their involvement in service development plans

(iv) additional services, which include contraceptive services, child health surveillance, vaccination and immunisation, maternity services, cervical cytology, and minor surgery

receptionists and practice nurses, few employ any additional staff. Other primary care staff are provided by the Health Services Executive (HSE) (see Chapter 11) but provision of other staff is still fairly sparse, with the notable exception of public health nurses – of whom there is quite a good network. Public health nurses fulfil the combined roles of health visitors and district nurses. They are qualified nurses with additional training and qualifications in public health nursing, and often also in midwifery and paediatric nursing.

The Health Services Executive also employs social workers, but their liaison with general practice and even public health nursing is often quite weak. Community pharmacists operate almost exclusively in commercial enterprises (chemist's shops). They have contracts with the Health Executive for the dispensing of medicines to patients under the GMS system (see Chapter 11) and the operation of the long-term illnesses and drug payment refund schemes. They have less involvement in medicine management with GPs than has become the case in the UK, though some are developing a medicine management role within nursing homes and other long-stay institutions.

Non-statutory/voluntary bodies, many of which have had traditional links to religious organisations, have extensive involvement in the provision of health and social care in Ireland. Many GPs make extensive use of the services they provide.

Further Reading

Caulfield E 2001 The organisation of the healthcare services in Ireland. A general practitioner's perspective. Irish College of General Practice, Dublin

Department of Health 2003 Investing in general practice, the new General Medical Services Contract. Department of Health, London

The GP in the healthcare system

The provision of health services is a major enterprise absorbing very substantial resources in virtually every country in the world. Most healthcare systems have workers who can be identified as having some, if not all, of the characteristics and functions of the general practitioner (see Chapter 1). However, where and how such a healthcare professional fits into the overall system for the provision of healthcare varies greatly.

At one end of the spectrum, as seen in many Scandinavian countries, family doctors are employees of a completely state funded and provided healthcare system, into which primary care is tightly integrated. At the other end of the spectrum, for instance in the USA, the role of general practitioner is fulfilled by a variety of doctors who provide their services on a commercial basis to the state, healthcare insurers and individuals. Contracts with payers vary greatly, from the fairly loose and broadly implied arrangements a doctor might have with individuals paying for themselves or their families to fairly tight arrangements with health maintenance organisations.

Other countries lie between these extremes. Many European countries have systems that are based on a mixture of state provision for the poor and healthcare insurance funded primary care for the rest of their citizens. The extent and influence of distinctive general practice or family medicine varies considerably. In many other parts of the world state involvement in general practice (as opposed to primary care) is minimal or non-existent and general practice, if it exists at all, is fairly weak.

The GP in the UK system

Brief history of the UK system

Prior to the establishment of the National Health Service (NHS) in 1948 most people were responsible for the cost of their own healthcare, both hospital and GP, although there were rudimentary arrangements under the Poor Law for the very poor to be cared for at the expense of local authorities. In 1911 Lloyd George introduced a national insurance scheme through which many working people could obtain healthcare for themselves (and sometimes their families) on payment of an insurance stamp on a regular basis rather than a fee at the time of a visit. GPs employed under this scheme were paid a capitation fee for each patient assigned to them and they saw patients in dispensaries. The rest of the population could see any doctor they chose but had to pay for their services at the point of delivery.

Wealthy people tended to consult specialists of their own choosing, while poorer people would avail of the services of GPs who sometimes, for the very poor, provided services without charge. Hospitals generally charged for their services, although poor people could sometimes be reimbursed for the cost of their care. In the latter part of the 19th century and the early 20th century there were an increasing number of voluntary and charitable hospitals, that sought to provide care at little or no direct cost to poorer patients, and an increasing range of municipal hospitals funded from local taxes.

With the institution of the NHS in 1948 people were provided access that was free at the point of use to all health services – both hospital and general practice – and paid for out of general taxation. At this time a clear separation arose between hospital doctors, who were becoming increasingly specialised and sub-specialised, and general practitioners, who operated primarily in the community. As part of ensuring this separation GPs were persuaded to forego admitting rights to hospitals in exchange for an exclusive right to see NHS patients in the community. Thus hospital and general practice came to be separated and GPs were placed in a clear gatekeeping role (see Chapter 8).

General practitioner services were extremely underdeveloped at the institution of the NHS and little improvement occurred in the succeeding two decades. GPs often operated out of poorly equipped premises with few, if any, ancillary staff. In 1966 a new charter for general practice was negotiated, through which GPs were able to obtain funding for improving their premises, employment of extra staff and general development of their services. GPs were also offered incentives to join into group practices. This led to a sustained trend towards the development of general practice and primary care in general.

In 1990 another new contract was introduced in UK general practice, which placed more emphasis on the development of preventive services. Greater accountability of GPs was also sought through the introduction of medical audit systems (see Chapters 5 and 6). A scheme, called indicative drug budgeting, was introduced. It rewarded GPs who stayed within predetermined drug spending targets by allowing them retain some of the putative 'savings' towards prescribed practice developments. In the 1990s GP fundholding was introduced whereby GPs could opt to control the budgets for many of the secondary care services for their patients. This was further developed in total purchasing schemes, where consortia of GPs could, working together, control the budget of the entirety of secondary and community care services.

A change in administration led to these schemes being abandoned but the value of having GPs centrally involved in the commissioning of care for their patients from other healthcare providers was appreciated – this element of these schemes was retained in the new structures introduced. In England, these were Primary Care Groups – groups of GPs and other primary care professionals who held budgets for other forms of healthcare provision – but these have now been supplanted by Primary Care Trusts (see below).

Administrative structure

Key features of the NHS are that it is a state funded system that aims to provide comprehensive healthcare (including primary, secondary and tertiary healthcare) to meet everyone's healthcare needs and is cost-free at the point of use. It is under the political responsibility of the Minister of Health (or equivalent in Scotland, Wales and Northern Ireland) but is overseen by the NHS Executive based in Leeds (or equivalents in other countries of the UK). It has traditionally been managed at a more local level by Health Authorities (or Health and Social Services Boards in the case of Scotland and Northern Ireland) – although in England Strategic Health Authorities and Primary Care Trusts have now supplanted these authorities.

Hospital services are mostly provided through NHS Acute Trusts, bodies responsible for the overall running and governance of single or multiple hospitals and/or other specialist services. GPs have traditionally been independent contractors who have contracted their services to the NHS under an arrangement known as General Medical Services (GMS). Since 1998 GPs (and, indeed, other primary care providers such as nurses) have been able to negotiate their own contract with the NHS, unrestrained by the provisions of the GMS, under an arrangement known as Personal Medical Services (PMS). An increasing number of GPs providing care under PMS arrangements are salaried rather than self-employed.

A new contract for general practitioners was introduced in the UK in 2004. While it retains some elements of the previous contract, being based on a mixture of capitation fees (i.e. an annual payment for each patient on the GP's list) and special allowances and payments for particular services, it is designed to allow practices greater flexibility in choosing the services they wish to provide. It also provides significant financial rewards for performance and clinical outcomes in a number of key areas. These key areas include practice organisation, preventive medicine (particularly cardiovascular disease), patient access and patient satisfaction.

Primary Care Trusts

Primary Care Trusts (PCTs) are statutory NHS bodies responsible for the provision of health services, including GP services, in a locality. They negotiate, in consultation with GPs in their area, contracts for the provision of services from Acute Trusts and other healthcare providers – sometimes including private healthcare providers. They provide GP services through contracts with GPs under either GMS or PMS arrangements, or occasionally by the direct provision of GP services through PMS schemes. They also control budgets for medicines prescribed by GPs in their area and assign prescribing budgets to GPs. GPs are expected to limit their prescribing to the amounts allocated to them through an annual drug budgeting process. PCTs, furthermore, are responsible for a wide range of other primary care services including:

- pharmacy services
- community nursing services
- dental health services
- optician and ophthalmological services
- NHS walk-in centres.

315

They are also expected to work closely with NHS Direct, a national telephone advice service for patients. PCTs are also charged with the task of clinical governance – a term used to describe systems and procedures designed to ensure that the service delivered to patients via the NHS is reasonably consistent throughout the system, is of high quality and is optimal in value-for-money terms. GPs are reasonably well represented on the Executive of PCTs under the rules governing the make up of the Trusts.

Position of the GP

As of September 2004 there were 31 523 GPs in England looking after an average of 1666 patients each. Of these, 37% were employed under PMS arrangements (see above) and the rest in GMS practices. They are in 8542 practices, of which 1918 are single-handed, i.e. have only one general practitioner principal. Most work in fairly large multidisciplinary teams with an average of 4.5 GPs and 10 whole-time equivalent practice staff, of whom nearly 75% are clerical and administrative staff and about 20% are practice nurses (Table 11.1). This does not include other nursing staff employed by the PCT.

GPs are ultimately responsible for the care they deliver personally and are vicariously responsible for much of the care delivered by others in the team. Thus GPs tend to be able to exert considerable influence on what care is delivered, and how and by whom it is delivered in respect of their registered populations. Furthermore, GPs control, to a considerable degree, patients' access to other health services – occupying a position often referred to as the 'gatekeeper' role (see Chapter 8). In recent times GPs in the UK have gone beyond traditional gatekeeping at the individual level and been given greater responsibility regarding the planning, delivery and strategic development of all health services, including hospital services, for populations. This role has evolved with the development of GP fundholding (see above), total purchasing schemes, locality commissioning and, most recently, through Primary Care Trusts.

Table 11.1
Numbers and proportions of practice staff employed by NHS principals (2004)

Practice staff type (whole-time equivalents)	Numbers	Percentage
Practice nurse	13563	18.8
Other direct patient-care providers	3591	5.0
Admin and clerical	53290	74.0
Other	561	2.2

From Statistics for General Medical Practitioners in England 1994–2004 from the UK Department of Health.

These are all expressions of the frequently restated desire of successive UK governments to develop a 'primary care led NHS' in which GPs are, at least theoretically, central to the provision and strategic development of the service. Being assigned this major role in allocation of NHS resources presents GPs with many challenges, including the ethical challenges discussed in Chapter 12.

The future of UK general practice

In 2000 the UK government published the National Health Services Plan, which maps out the future envisioned for the NHS. It commits the government to a substantial investment of extra resources in the NHS but it also seeks to implement major reforms in how health services are delivered. Thus, there is a commitment to increase the number of GPs by 2000 and to modernise 3000 practice premises – including the construction of 250 new primary care centres. The more quality focused, locally negotiated, flexible and accountable Personal Medical Services arrangements will be promoted and will, to a large extent, replace the traditional GMS system (see New GMS Contract, below). Single-handed practice, in particular, will be given extra attention with regard to quality assurance – special arrangements for clinical governance of single-handed practice are anticipated.

An increased role for other primary care professionals, especially nurses and pharmacists, is also to be enabled and encouraged. This will, inevitably, lead to changes in the roles fulfilled by GPs. For example, nurses will be able to assume some of the burden of looking after minor illnesses and play a greater role in chronic disease management while pharmacists may have a more active role in the monitoring and regulation of repeat prescriptions.

The NHS Plan also promises the development of new mental health professionals who will be able to relieve GPs of some of the work of looking after people with psychological problems. GPs in their turn will be expected to specialise more, developing extra knowledge and skills in certain disease areas and then becoming a source of expertise to other GPs – allowing more patients to receive more of their care in the primary care setting. Consultants, too, will be encouraged to do outreach work with the larger primary care centres, to bring care closer to patients.

Other major planks of the NHS Plan are a greater amount of patient involvement in service design and development and greater accountability of service providers. These will place new pressures on GPs to demonstrate the value of their work to outside scrutiny. A major area of concern in the current NHS is waiting times in general practice. There is a commitment to reduce these so patients will be guaranteed access to a primary care professional within 24 hours and to a primary care doctor within 48 hours. Some of this improvement may be enabled by further developments of NHS Direct, the national telephone service for health advice. This will become a one-stop shop for all patient contact with NHS providers and will also be available online. Patients will be able to seek advice, get test results and book appointments with their GP via NHS Direct over the telephone or via e-mail.

A further evolution envisaged is that health and social services will come together under one organisational structure in Care Trusts. Both health and social services are already under one authority in Scotland and Northern Ireland, so this development will bring England and Wales in line. This should facilitate closer working of GPs and other primary healthcare workers with social services – reducing problems of inter-agency working that are particularly acute with older patients.

The NHS Plan is clearly an ambitious one that, even if only partially realised, will have major implications for how GPs work, although the core tasks of GPs and the singular importance of their relationships with their patients are likely to be retained whatever happens.

The new General Medical Services contract

In 2004 a new contract for the provision of general medical services was implemented in the UK. This contract is effectively the implementation of key primary care aspects of the NHS Plan (see above). The responsibility for the provision of general medical services now rests with primary care organisations (PCOs) – typically Primary Care Trusts. The

PCOs will usually contract with practices for certain basic services for registered patients. They may also contract with practices for other additional and enhanced services and out-of-hours services but, particularly where practices opt out of providing these services, the PCO may also contract with other providers. PCOs may also provide services themselves by employing GPs (as opposed to contracting with them) and providing what are referred to as Personal Medical Services (PMS).

The quality and outcomes of primary care services will be ascertained through a mechanism called the Quality and Outcomes Framework (QOF). The QOF has four main domains, the clinical, organisational and additional services, and the patient experience. Some details of the clinical aspects of the QOF are covered in Chapter 5; other details of the QOF are discussed in Chapter 10. The patient experience aspects of the contract relate to patient satisfaction (to be ascertained in regular patient satisfaction surveys) and consultation length. Practices will be rewarded financially for achievement of agreed targets within the QOF. In addition, a large investment in information technology has been put in place to allow for monitoring of performance under this very elaborate contract. Time will tell if this innovative approach to practice development achieves its goals.

The GP in the Irish system

Brief history of the Irish system

Until the founding of the Irish state in 1921 its healthcare system was the same as that of the rest of the United Kingdom. Thus Ireland inherited the dispensary system of general practitioner services and the mixture of private, voluntary, charitable and municipal hospitals that already existed – along with the general system of most people having to provide for their own healthcare. When the NHS was founded in the UK there was a debate in Ireland about whether or not a similar system should be introduced. It was decided against, although a limited scheme to provide free healthcare for expectant mothers and their children (the Mother and Infant Scheme, see below) was introduced.

The existing dispensary system was gradually developed to look after the GP healthcare needs of the poorest in society. Hospitals were funded to an ever-increasing extent by the state to provide care free at the point of use for up to two-thirds of the population. Some 60% of the population remained responsible for the cost of their own GP care and 30% for the cost their hospital care – although there was a government subsidised healthcare insurance scheme to cover the costs of hospital care.

A review of GP services in the late 1960s led to the abolition of the dispensary system and its replacement by the General Medical Services (GMS) scheme. Under this scheme, known colloquially as the 'choice of doctor' scheme, families deemed unable to afford to provide their own healthcare were issued with medical cards, entitling them to register with the GP of their choice and obtain medicines at no cost. GPs were obliged to treat patients seeking assistance under the GMS exactly as they would treat all their other patients. Initially, GPs in the scheme were paid a standard fee for each patient visit or service provided but in the late 1980s this fee-per-item system was replaced with a capitation system (see below).

Administrative structures

Healthcare in Ireland is funded through a mixture of public and private funding, with approximately 75% from general taxation and the remainder through direct payment by patients – who may be able to recoup some or all of the cost from health insurers. Secondary care is provided by public hospitals, voluntary hospitals (largely state funded but enjoying a degree of autonomy from state control) and private hospitals. Although everyone is now entitled to free hospital care (excluding Accident and Emergency if self-referred), about one-third of the population has health insurance and generally uses private healthcare. About one-third of the population is eligible for state funded (public) GP services through the General Medical Services scheme (GMS), with the rest paying their GP directly at the time of accessing the service. Of these, a small proportion, on the more expensive insurance plans, may be eligible for a refund from their insurer.

Overall political responsibility for healthcare resides with the legislature and the government, within which health is looked after by the Department of Health and Children. Since 2005 day-to-day running of the service has been the responsibility of the Health Services Executive (HSE), with the Department setting policy and planning strategic direction only. The HSE has two major directorates – one for acute hospitals and one for primary, continuing, and community care (PCCC). The PCCC directorate operates through four regional offices and 32 local health offices. These arrangements replace the 11 health boards previously responsible for the running of the health services.

The General Medical Services scheme

The General Medical Services (GMS) scheme was introduced in 1970 to replace the dispensary scheme (see above). The main determinant of a person's eligibility for GP services under this scheme is income. Eligible patients include:

- people with incomes below certain thresholds (usually determined on an annual basis)
- people dependent exclusively on state benefits
- people with no incomes such as refugees and asylum seekers.

Most GMS patients also receive all medicines prescribed by their doctors for free – although since 2005 there is a category of cardholder who only receives GP services for free. Local Health Offices have limited discretion to provide medical cards to other people who do not meet the income eligibility criteria but who have other special needs (such as serious long-term illnesses or disabilities). Under the terms of the scheme, doctors are paid an annual capitation fee for each patient registered with them – the amount of the fee varying with the age and gender of the patient.

In addition, GPs are paid fees for the provision of certain additional services including out-of-hours visits, minor operations, nebulisation of people with asthma etc. GPs in the scheme are also able to recoup part of the cost of employing certain practice staff. They are, however, expected to restrict the costs of medicines prescribed to within a budget set annually. They are rewarded for doing so by becoming eligible for practice development monies, which will be refunded to them if used to enhance their practices in certain specified ways.

Other schemes for GP services

In addition to the GMS there are a number of other schemes whereby patients can have access to certain GP services funded by the State. The Mother and Child Scheme provides for antenatal and postnatal care of mothers and their babies free at the point of use and for which GPs, deemed suitably qualified, are remunerated by the State. The Primary Immunisation Scheme also provides appropriate patients access to free primary vaccinations, according to government immunisation policy. The necessary vaccines are provided free and GPs are paid for administering the vaccines – and may be eligible for additional payments for the achievement of certain population immunisation coverage targets.

The Methadone Maintenance Programme reimburses GPs who undertake the supervision of patients on methadone maintenance programmes initiated by the drug abuse treatment services. The number of patients a given GP may supervise under the scheme and the level of remuneration received are related to the level of specified training the GP will have undertaken to become eligible for the scheme.

The position of the GP

GPs in Ireland operate mostly as either single-handed GPs or in small groups of two or three – larger groups do exist but are less common (see Table 11.2). They tend to work in small teams with receptionists and practice nurses being fairly common but the number of these in each practice is generally low. Other types of staff are rare (see Table 11.3 and Chapter 10).

GPs in Ireland function as 'gatekeepers' to other (secondary) services, particularly within the public health sector –

Table 11.2
Numbers of GPs in Irish practices

Number of partners	Number of GPs	Percentage
Single-handed	823	42
2 partners	559	28
3 partners	302	15
4 or more	289	14

From Caulfield E 2001 The organisation of the healthcare services in Ireland. A general practitioner's perspective. Irish College of General Practice, Dublin.

Table 11.3
Numbers and proportions of staff employed in Irish GP practices

Staff type	Number	Percent of practices employing
Secretaries	791	47
Receptionists	415	24
Nurses	389	25
Managers	46	4
Other	94	6

From Caulfield E 2001 The organisation of the healthcare services in Ireland. A general practitioner's perspective. Irish College of General Practice, Dublin.

and to a considerable extent within the private sector, too. GPs have only limited access to and influence on the decision-making processes controlling the health services. There are also GPs appointed, mostly on a part-time basis, to Primary Care units to advise these units on GP matters. Local faculties of the Irish College of General Practitioners and branches of the Irish Medical Organisation (the representative body and trade union for most GPs) are also consulted on a regular basis about local health policies and initiatives. The corresponding national bodies also confer regularly with the Department of Health and Children on GP matters.

The future of Irish general practice

In 2001 the Irish government published a primary health-care strategy. This is a major development in strategic thinking on Irish healthcare regarding the importance of primary care to the overall system. The key feature is the development of larger and more integrated primary care teams. The basic model would comprise 4–5 GPs working closely with a similar number of nurses, a slightly larger number of administrative staff and a number of other health and social care professionals – including care assistants, physiotherapists, occupational therapists and social workers. These teams will be based in single well-designed and modern premises. The idea is that such teams would be able to work in a more cohesive way than these professionals currently do and would be able to unburden the secondary care services of some of the routine work of caring for people – especially those with chronic health problems.

These primary care teams would, in turn, be able to draw on the support of a wider range of health and social care professionals organised in 'primary care networks'. These would include pharmacists, chiropodists, speech and language therapists, dieticians and so on. These teams and networks would be better equipped than before with improved information and communications technology, which should also enhance communications between the different sectors and promote more 'seamless' healthcare. Patients would be encouraged to enrol with local primary healthcare teams and have open access to consult with any member of the team without the need for formal referral. Voluntary enrolment of patients should facilitate more effective delivery of preventive services – which are currently rather haphazardly provided in the Irish system.

Other elements of the strategy envisage major investments in both infrastructure and personnel in primary care, the further development of more effective out-of-hours arrangements, the development of a national telephone patient access and advice service (similar to NHS Direct in the UK) and the development of academic primary care centres. The basic administrative and consultative structures to begin to develop the plan are now in place, as of

2005, but the major investment programme has not yet materialised.

Further Reading

Caulfield E 2001 The organisation of the healthcare services in Ireland. A general practitioner's perspective. Irish College of General Practice, Dublin

Department of Health 2000 The NHS plan. A plan for investment, a plan for reform. The Stationery Office, London

Department of Health 2003 Investing in general practice, the new General Medical Services Contract. Department of Health, London

Department of Health and Children 2001 Primary care. A new direction. The Stationery Office, Dublin

12

Ethical aspects of general practice

Ethical issues arise in general practice just as they do in all branches of medical practice. Many of the momentous issues of medical ethics, such as those surrounding the beginning and end of life (abortion, infertility, brain death, euthanasia and so on), do arise occasionally in general practice. However, the practice of medicine by GPs is characterised by many seemingly more minor ethical issues on a day-to-day basis. These 'micro-ethical' decisions require no less skill and judgement in their resolution, although the consequences of misjudgement may be apparently less grave. Recognising the ethical aspects of everyday decisions and applying sound ethical principles to them should improve the quality and morality of decisions made and, thus, patient care.

There are several important frameworks used for making ethical decisions (see Box 12.1), of which the deontological principles of benevolence (doing the most good), non-maleficence (doing the least harm), justice and autonomy are probably the most widely applied in medical ethical decision-making including in general practice. How ethical thinking and decision-making are applied in general practice is illustrated below with reference to some of the ethical dilemmas commonly faced by GPs.

Box 12.1   Frameworks for ethical decision-making

- Utilitarianism
- Obligation-based ethics – Kantian
- Virtue-based ethics
- Rights-based ethics
- Communitarianism
- Relational ethics
- Case-based ethics – Casuistry
- Principal-based ethics – Deontological

Informed consent

All medical diagnosis and treatment should be undertaken only with the informed consent of the patient. This is a basic requirement arising out of the principle of respect for patient autonomy. In general practice, consent to diagnostic manoeuvres and treatment is usually assumed to exist on the basis that voluntary attendance at the doctor's surgery is an indication of 'implied consent' – i.e. the act of going to a doctor implies that you consent to what doctors normally do. It is not always clear exactly how far implied consent can be taken to apply and when explicit consent should be sought instead. In other branches of medicine explicit consent is sought where the dangers of diagnostic or therapeutic interventions are deemed to be high.

Though grave danger to life or limb is rare in general practice there are situations where consent is best not assumed but should be sought explicitly. For example, history taking involving asking questions about sensitive issues such as sexuality could be difficult or intrusive for the patient. In such situations explicit verbal consent to be asked about certain issues should be sought before asking them. Likewise, permission for intimate examinations ought to be obtained explicitly and verbally before proceeding.

Explicit written consent is rarely required in general practice but should be sought before unusual procedures such as video or audio recording of consultations (such as might be done for training or research purposes) or for potentially risky, even if minor, surgical procedures.

Explicit consent to prescribe a treatment for a patient is not usually required in general practice but the other important aspect of informed consent, namely to ensure that the patient is adequately informed about treatment being offered, is an important requirement of ethical treatment (see also Chapter 7 on information that should be provided to patients about their medicines).

GPs often take blood tests and order other investigations on patients. None of these is without risk and the patient's informed consent should be explicitly sought. The doctor must know enough about the investigations to adequately inform the patient and then seek consent. The information provided to patients regarding tests should include:

- the name of the test
- what is involved in having the test
- the risks of the test
- the risks of not having the test
- what might be discovered by the test
- what can/will be done depending on the results of the test.

However, as many tests in the general practice setting are being used to rule out serious disease rather than necessarily prove a diagnosis (see Chapter 2) the GP may have to exercise caution in how much to tell the patient about what the test is for – in order to reduce the risk of harm to the patient from stimulating unnecessary alarm. It is, though, probably better to err on the side of telling the patient more as the ethic of respecting the patient autonomy is coming to be perceived (by patients and their representatives, at least) as more important than keeping the patient from the potential harm of worrying unnecessarily (i.e. the ethic of non-maleficence that has informed the paternalism of traditional medical ethics).

Confidentiality

All doctors are governed by an ethical duty to keep in confidence information given by patients. Maintaining this can be particularly challenging in general practice, where a doctor may deal with many members of the same family or people who have other relationships with the patient that makes them feel entitled to information about that patient. It can seem churlish and unnecessarily obstructive for a GP to refuse to discuss the care of a person with their spouse, or of an elderly person with their relatives. Indeed, it is often impractical to maintain a stance of complete non-disclosure with relatives about each other's health care. Often they will have divulged information to relatives anyway. However, GPs should be alert to how easily confidentiality is broken in family practice or in a community setting.

Information about patients should not be discussed with non-relatives without the patient's explicit consent. Even with relatives you need to have a good idea of what the relationship is between people and the state of that relationship before sharing any information. The best, but not always practicable, policy is only to discuss patient care with relatives in the presence of the patient. GPs, who are responsible for the actions of their staff, must ensure that all staff are aware of the need for absolute patient confidentiality. Staff should receive adequate training and contracts of employment should make clear the serious consequences of any breach of confidentiality, however inadvert.

Truth telling

Respect for the patient's autonomy also demands that doctors tell their patients the truth. However, it is not always as simple as telling the patient the whole truth all the time. The whole truth at the wrong time can have harmful consequences that might outweigh any benefits. Breaking bad news to patients is an area of general practice where the issues of truth telling come to the fore (see also Chapter 9).

The first step in breaking bad news is to be alert to the patient's possible reactions to hearing an unfavourable diagnosis. If you can identify that a patient may interpret some information about their health as bad, do not hide the information but take extra care about when and how the truth is conveyed. A good general principle is that you should never wilfully lie to patients but there may be occasions where a delay in telling the full truth can be the compassionate and ethical way to proceed.

When it comes to telling patients what might be painful truths it is often better to let patients decide the rate and explicitness of disclosure. Thus, patients with incurable cancer may be asked what they would like to know about their condition. They may want to know only whether or not it is 'bad', whether they are 'going to get better', or whether or not it is cancer/malignant. Even if patients ask if it is a specific diagnosis like 'cancer' this does not mean they are ready to receive the full picture with regard to treatment or prognosis. You should endeavour to break bad news in a gentle and timely way (out of the duty to do no harm), while not holding back, distorting, or denying the truth (out of respect for patient autonomy).

Euthanasia, assisted suicide and withdrawal of treatment

The conditions which give rise to requests from patients to their doctors to either end their lives or assist them in taking their own lives are relatively rare, yet most GPs will receive such requests several times in a professional lifetime. In countries where euthanasia is legally provided for, such as the Netherlands, GPs have a pivotal role in ensuring that the legal guidelines for such actions are followed. They also have a role in carrying out any euthanasia procedure.

In the UK the consensus still prevails that doctors must not participate in acts of euthanasia or assisted suicide, regardless of any patient's request. This stance is informed, in part, by the generally held view among specialists in the care of the dying (i.e. palliative care doctors) that there are always ways in which patients can be helped. Suffering can always be reduced, and thus it is always unnecessary to invoke euthanasia as a solution to the patient's problem.

Euthanasia must be distinguished from death that may result as a side effect of treatment given for reasons other than to deliberately end the patient's life. Euthanasia is a deliberate act, undertaken with the express purpose of ending the patient's life. Actions that lead to death but for which bringing about the death was not the intended outcome do not constitute euthanasia.

Where a treatment, given for its beneficial effect, leads to the patient's demise as an undesirable effect, it may be considered to be ethically acceptable as long as one's goal is to achieve the desirable effect and the desirable effect is not achieved through the harmful effect. This is known as the 'rule of double effect'. An example of this is where a dose of morphine is given to a terminally ill patient, even though that dose might prove fatal – as long as the dose is given for the purpose of relieving pain or suffering the fatal effect does not constitute euthanasia.

A more common scenario is where a patient is terminally ill and decisions have to be made regarding treatments to be instituted or withdrawn. A useful rule of thumb for this situation is that, as long as death is clearly the inevitable final outcome of the patient's illness, treatments should be instituted only where they contribute to the patient's comfort. In other words, one is not obliged to 'strive officiously' to keep the patient alive, and indeed it could be unethical to initiate a treatment that is likely to be futile. In patients in a terminal condition fluids and nutrition would normally be maintained but a supervening pneumonia might not be treated, especially if this is more likely to prolong the process of dying rather than really prolong the patient's life.

Decisions are often difficult in these situations and you should seek advice from specialists (such as palliative care doctors), from colleagues (including nursing and other non-medical colleagues), and from the patient and relatives where appropriate.

Assessing physical and mental capacity

There are many situations in which doctors are asked to assess the physical or mental capacity of their patients. These nearly always pose some ethical difficulties for the doctor. Sickness certification is one such area. Doctors, especially general practitioners, are charged by society with determining the legitimacy of people's claim to be ill. Being ill brings with it certain dispensations from ordinary duties and may also entitle you to claim state benefits. Doctors are asked to apply the ethical principle of justice to ensure that people do not obtain these benefits at the expense of others unjustly or unfairly. However, doctors are also obliged by their duty of respecting their patients' autonomy to advocate for their patients and ensure they get their due entitlements.

Often these judgements are relatively straightforward because most illness claims are quite legitimate. However, it can be more problematic if a patient asks to be signed off sick for, say, social reasons (e.g. to look after another ill person) when they are not, in fact, discernibly ill. While you may have some sympathy for the patient's plight, you cannot certify them as ill when they are not.

An even trickier situation can arise with older people seeking a certificate of medical fitness to drive. The ability to drive is an important facet of the wellbeing of many elderly. It allows them to get out and go places which, if they were denied this, might render them housebound, depressed and, ultimately, more seriously ill. However, the requirements for older people to be re-certified as fit to drive have been placed there for the protection of all road users, including the older persons themselves. People could be hurt or killed in any accident resulting from any significant impairment in the capacity to drive of an elderly patient.

Assessing the mental capacity of patients arises less frequently, but when it does it poses major ethical issues. One of the potential consequences of certain mental incapacities can be the involuntary loss of liberty. This is a major affront to a person's autonomy. Where it is judged that a mentally ill patient is a danger to others, there is a conflict between the common good of society, which impinges on doctors as their duty to behave justly, and the autonomy of the patient. Where patients are judged to be a danger to themselves, the dilemma is between the duty to the maximum good for the patients (beneficence) and the duty to respect the patients' autonomy. If it is decided patients do have an illness sufficiently dangerous to need involuntary admission, they have only temporarily impaired autonomy and should still be afforded all the respect and dignity due to anyone who is compos mentis.

Another area where GPs may be called upon to assess mental capacity is when a patient is making or has made a will or other legal transactions. Here matters may be more straightforward ethically, because your duty is clearly to the patient. If in your best judgement you decide the patient is compos mentis then the patient will retain control of any personal business, which would be what, no doubt, they would want. If you decide patients are not sufficiently well mentally to look after their affairs then it is in their best interests that someone else be appointed to do so. Either way, as long as the doctor's clinical judgement is not flawed, the patient is best served by whatever ensues.

Resource allocation

The formal involvement of GPs in the allocation of healthcare resources through such initiatives as fundholding and now Primary Care Trusts is relatively new (see Chapter 11). GPs, though, like all healthcare professionals, allocate resources to patients every time they interact with them. Time given to patients, prescriptions issued to patients, investigations ordered for patients and referrals of patients to others all end up consuming resources which, once allocated to one patient, may not be available for others. This is the concept of 'opportunity cost'. Recent UK government initiatives, such as healthcare commissioning by GPs and drug budgeting (see Chapter 7), are really just ways of making these resource allocation decisions and their consequences elsewhere in the system more explicit to GPs and their patients.

The distribution of resources needs to be governed by ethical principles, particularly those of justice or fairness. However, allocating resources fairly is not that easy, even if that is the clear goal. A major difficulty lies in deciding what constitutes fairness in this context. Should healthcare resources be distributed equally, or according to need, or according to capacity to benefit, or on some other basis?

An equal distribution of healthcare resources with everyone being given exactly the same makes no sense as there is little need to expend healthcare resources on the healthy when there are ill people to be looked after. However, variations on the principles of everyone getting an equal share give rise to concepts such as the 'fair opportunity rule', which suggests that everyone should have equal access to healthcare regardless of other factors such as race, gender, intelligence or age. While few would have problems with these ideas conceptually, there is ample evidence that our healthcare system is not equally accessible to everyone. This implies that the ethical principle of equity is being breached.

There are other issues, too – particularly if you consider people of different ages. While you might feel that older people should not be denied access to healthcare on the basis of their age alone, it may be proposed that some healthcare resources, such as coronary artery bypass, be made available to younger patients before older patients. This must be done on grounds of perceived capacity to benefit or likely total benefit to the individuals rather than purely on age grounds. To do otherwise would be ageist – and unethical.

The obvious grounds for distributing healthcare resources are on the basis of medical need but there are difficulties in determining what is need, as opposed to want or demand. Furthermore, there are also ethical issues surrounding who should make these decisions – doctors, patients or managers? Do patients' requests for treatments for infertility, or erectile dysfunction, or male-pattern baldness or cosmetic surgery constitute medical wants or medical needs? Even if it is agreed that someone has a medical need, people's different needs must be prioritised because not all needs can be met within the resources available.

One reasonable ground on which to adjudicate between competing medical needs relates to capacity to benefit, i.e. that medical resources would be expended preferentially on those who would gain the most from any medical intervention. This approach still leaves problems with ascertaining how beneficial a given intervention will be in a given patient and questions of how to compare different kinds of benefits – such as years of life gained compared with quality of life gained.

Allocation of resources within the healthcare system is an ethically very taxing area, even for experts. GPs, who are increasingly becoming involved in these difficult decisions in quite an explicit and high level way, need to appreciate the ethical issues involved and seek guidance from others in resolving the many ethical issues that will arise.

Further Reading

Dowrick C, Frith L (eds) 1999 General practice and ethics. Uncertainty and responsibility. Routledge, London

Orme-Smith A, Spicer J 2001 Ethics in general practice. A practical handbook for personal development. Radcliffe Medical Press, Oxford

Rogers W, Braunack-Mayer A 2004 Practical ethics for general practice. Oxford University Press, Oxford

Index